FORENSIC PATHOLOGY

A Handbook For
Pathologists

Edited By

RUSSELL S. FISHER, M.D.

CHARLES S. PETTY, M.D.

This project was supported by Grant Number NI 71-118G awarded to the College of American Pathologists by the National Institute of Law Enforcement and Criminal Justice, Law Enforcement Assistance Administration, U.S. Department of Justice, under the Omnibus Crime Control and Safe Streets Act of 1968, as amended. Points of view or opinions stated in this document are those of the contributors and do not necessarily represent the official position or policies of the U.S. Department of Justice.

July 1977

National Institute of Law Enforcement and Criminal Justice
Law Enforcement Assistance Administration
U. S. Department of Justice

For sale by the Superintendent of Documents, U.S. Government Printing Office
Washington, D.C. 20402
Stock Number 027–000–00541–1

CONTENTS

CONTRIBUTORS

Michael M. Baden, M.D.
Deputy Chief Medical Examiner
City of New York
Associate Professor of Forensic Medicine
New York University School of Medicine
New York, New York

John F. Burton, M.D.
Chief Medical Examiner
Oakland County
Pontiac, Michigan

Frank P. Cleveland, M.D.
Coroner of Hamilton County
Director, Institute of Forensic Medicine, Toxicology and Criminalistics
Associate Professor of Forensic Pathology
University of Cincinnati College of Medicine
Cincinnati, Ohio

John I. Coe, M.D.
Chief Medical Examiner
Hennepin County
Professor of Pathology
University of Minnesota Medical School
Chief of Pathology
Hennepin County General Hospital
Minneapolis, Minnesota

William G. Eckert, M.D.
Deputy Coroner
Sedgwich County
Adjunct Professor of Forensic Sciences
Wichita State University
Wichita, Kansas

John F. Edland, M.D.
Chief Medical Examiner
Monroe County
Clinical Associate Professor of Pathology
University of Rochester School of Medicine and Dentistry
Clinical Assistant Professor of Psychiatry
University of Rochester School of Medicine and Dentistry
Rochester, New York

Russell S. Fisher, M.D.
Chief Medical Examiner
State of Maryland
Clinical Professor of Forensic Pathology
University of Maryland School of Medicine
Associate in Forensic Pathology
Johns Hopkins University School of Hygiene and Public Health
Lecturer in Forensic Pathology
Johns Hopkins University School of Medicine
Baltimore, Maryland

Jerry T. Francisco, M.D.
Chief Medical Examiner
State of Tennessee
County Medical Examiner
Shelby County
Professor of Pathology and Director of Forensic Pathology
University of Tennessee College of Medicine
Memphis, Tennessee

Charles S. Hirsch, M.D.
Associate Pathologist and Deputy Coroner
Cuyahoga County Coroner's Office
Assistant Professor of Forensic Pathology
Case Western Reserve University School of Medicine
Cleveland, Ohio

George S. Loquvam, M.D.
Forensic Pathologist to Coroner
Alameda County
Lecturer in Forensic Medicine
Hastings School of Law
San Francisco
Lecturer in Forensic Medicine
Boalt Hall School of Law
Berkeley
Director, Institute of Forensic Sciences
Oakland, California

Leslie I. Lukash, M.D.
Chief Medical Examiner
Nassau County
Professor of Forensic Pathology
State University of New York at Stony Brook
East Meadow, New York

Arthur J. McBay, Ph.D.
Chief Toxicologist
State of North Carolina
Professor of Pathology
University of North Carolina School of Medicine
Professor of Pharmacy
University of North Carolina School of Pharmacy
Chapel Hill, North Carolina

FOREWORD

This publication represents an effort on the part of the College of American Pathologists to provide the community pathologist with basic information in the performance of the medical legal autopsy.

The development of the manual was made possible in part through funds provided by the National Institute of Law Enforcement and Criminal Justice of the LEAA. The major portion of the funding was used to conduct 13 seminars in Forensic Pathology attended by more than 350 community pathologists.

The authors of these chapters are all eminently qualified in the field of Forensic Medicine and the College extends to them a grateful thank you for their dedication and efforts to this project.

The material presented in this Handbook is not intended to serve as a substitute for existing publications, rather it is intended to serve as an additional source of information to assist the pathologist in meeting a community responsibility.

The proper performance of the medical legal autopsy and the objective presentation of the findings is a public responsibility which has been accepted by many pathologists in this country.

It is the hope of the college that this publication will assist you in continuing your work in this area.

Robert Horn, M.D., *President,*
College of American Pathologists

PREFACE BY EDITORS

Our work was easy. We had a fine group of experts in the very broad field of pathology who did the majority of the work in writing this manual. We have tried to preserve the flavor of each person's style of writing. A few notes have been added to explain different points of view, but the content of the chapters represents the viewpoint of the individual authors.

Our goal was easy. We wanted to help make available to pathologists a workbook small enough to be packed in the bag with the autopsy instruments; short enough to make it possible to review any given chapter prior to (or during) an autopsy.

We give it to you—the patologists.

We hope you find it useful—and use it.

Russell S. Fisher, M.D.   Charles S. Petty, M.D.
Baltimore, Maryland   Dallas, Texas

Chapter I

FORENSIC AUTOPSY PROCEDURE

Leslie I. Lukash, M.D.
Chief Medical Examiner
Nassau County, New York

Introduction, Concepts and Principles

It is assumed that all pathologists know the construction and requirements for reporting the findings of a complete postmortem examination. The following is a guide for use in converting the standard autopsy protocol into the report of a medicolegal autopsy. All of the usual descriptive technics should be maintained. Greater attention to detail, accurate description of abnormal findings, and the addition of final conclusions and interpretations, will bring about this transformation.

The **hospital autopsy** is an examination performed with the consent of the deceased person's relatives for the purposes of: (1) determining the cause of death; (2) providing correlation of clinical diagnosis and clinical symptoms; (3) determining the effectiveness of therapy; (4) studying the natural course of disease processes; and (5) educating students and physicians.

The **medicolegal autopsy** is an examination performed under the law, usually ordered by the Medical Examiner and Coroner [1] for the purposes of: (1) determining the cause, manner,[2] and time of death; (2) recovering, identifying, and preserving evidentiary material; (3) providing interpretation and correlation of facts and circumstances related to death; (4) providing a factual, objective medical report for law enforcement, prosecution, and defense agencies; and (5) separating death due to disease from death due to external causes for protection of the innocent.

The essential features of a medicolegal autopsy are: (1) to perform a complete autopsy; (2) to personally perform the examination and observe all findings so that interpretation may be sound; (3) to perform a thorough examination and overlook nothing which could later prove of importance; (4) to preserve all information by written and photographic records; and (5) to provide a professional report without bias.

---

[1] Editors note: In some jurisdictions the health officer, district attorney or others may order an autopsy.

[2] Editors note: Sometimes referred to as "mode" of death.

1

Preliminary Procedures

Before the clothing is removed, the body should be examined to determine the condition of the clothing, and to correlate tears and other defects with obvious injuries to the body, and to record the findings. The clothing, body, and hands should be protected from possible contamination prior to specific examination of each. A record of the general condition of the body and of the clothing should be made and the extent of rigor and lividity, the temperature of the body and the environment, and any other data pertinent to the subsequent determination of the time of death also should be recorded.

After the preliminary examination the clothing may be carefully removed by unbuttoning, unzippering, or unhooking to remove without tearing or cutting. If the clothing is wet or bloody, it must be hung up to dry in the air to prevent putrefaction and disintegration. Record and label each item of clothing. Preserve with proper identification for subsequent examination. Clothing may be examined in the laboratory with soft tissue x-ray and infrared photographs in addition to various chemical analyses and immunohematologic analyses.

Autopsy Procedure

The date, time and place of autopsy should be succinctly noted, and where and by whom it was performed, and any observers or participants should be named. The body should be identified, and all physical characteristics should be described. These include age, height, weight, sex, color of hair and eyes, state of nutrition and muscular development, scars, and tattoos. Description of the teeth, the number present and absent, and the general condition should be detailed noting any abnormalities or deformities, or evidence of fracture, old or recent. In a separate paragraph or paragraphs describe all injuries, noting the number and characteristics of each including size, shape, pattern, and location in relation to anatomic landmarks. Describe the course, direction, and depth of injuries and enumerate structures involved by the injury. Identify and label any foreign object recovered and specify its relation to a given injury.

At least one photograph should be taken to identify the body. Photograph injuries to document their location and be certain to include a scale to show their size. Photographs can be used to demonstrate and correlate external injuries with internal injuries and to demonstrate pathologic processes other than those of traumatic origin.

Roentgenographic and fluoroscopic examinations can be used to locate bullets or other radio-opaque objects, to identify the victim, and to document fractures, anatomic deformities, and surgical procedures when such metallic foreign bodies as plates, nails, screws, and wire sutures have been used.

A general description of the head, neck, cervical spine, thorax, abdo-

2

men, genitalia, and extremities should be given in logical sequence. The course of wounds through various structures should be detailed remembering variations of position in relationships during life versus relationships after death and when supine on the autopsy table. Evidentiary items such as bullets, knives, or portions thereof, pellets or foreign materials, should be preserved and the point of recovery should be noted. Each should be labelled for proper identification. Each organ should be dissected and described, noting relationships and conditions.

Special Examinations and Dissection Technics

Head. First examine the exterior of the scalp for injury hidden by the hair and the interior of the scalp for evidence of trauma not visible externally. Note the course and extent of fractures. When removing the calvarium keep the dura intact (subdural hemorrhage can thus be preserved for measurements). Strip dura from the calvarium to expose any fractures. Use a dental chart to specifically identify each tooth, its condition, the extent of caries and location of fillings.[3] Note the absence of any teeth. Examine both the upper and lower eyelids for petechial hemorrhages and the eyes for hidden wounds. Examine the ear canals for evidence of hemorrhage indicative of fracture. Examine the interior of the mouth, lips, and cheeks for evidence of trauma.

Neck. External examination of the neck should include observation of all aspects for contusions, abrasions, or petechiae. Manual strangulation is often characterized by a series of linear or curved abrasions and contusions. Ligature strangulation is characterized by a linear abrasion and some ligatures may produce definitive patterned abrasions. Ligature strangulation generally produces linear abrasion in a horizontal plane. Hanging characteristically produces a deep grooved abrasion with an inverted "V" at the point of suspension and a pattern may also be produced. Indistinct or obscure external injuries may become more apparent at completion of autopsy after blood has drained and the tissues begin to dry. For internal examination of the neck dissect the chest flap upward to the level of the chin, expose the neck muscles and organs after the neck vessels have been drained of blood by removal of the heart. Note the location of hemorrhage into muscles. Hemorrhage will be greatest in manual strangulation or severe blunt trauma of the neck. Remove the neck organs intact including the tongue. Dissect with extreme care so as not to break the hyoid bone during removal and dissect the muscles from the bone. Hemorrhage will be noted at the site of fracture. Thyroid or cricoid cartilages may also be fractured in manual strangulation and hemorrhage will be noted at the site of these fractures. The mucosa of the larynx, pyriform sinuses, and esophagus may show petechiae or hemorrhage. Examine the cervical spine anteriorly

---

[3] Editors note: In those cases where dental description is of crucial importance, a dentist may be of great assistance.

3

for hemorrhage in the muscles along the vertebrae. Hemorrhage will be present at the site of fractures of the cervical vertebrae. When vertebrae C-1 and C-2 are fractured dissection should be carried out from the posterior approach. The characteristic signs of asphyxia are cyanosis, petechiae in the conjunctivae, sclerae, eyelids, face, neck, upper chest, and internally in the pericardium, epicardium, and pleurae.

Cervical and thoracic spine. The cervical spine may be examined anteriorly or posteriorly. High cervical injuries are best demonstrated by the posterior approach. The thoracic spine may be readily examined from the interior (anterior) approach. Identify the specific injured vertebrae. Note any fracture, dislocation, compression, or evidence of hemorrhage at the site. Dissect the soft tissue and muscle from the surface in order to view the vertebral bodies. Small projectiles may enter vertebrae by splitting fibers and leave little obvious evidence of entrance. Open the spinal canal. Remove the cord to demonstrate any injury.

Chest. Detail fractures of ribs. Cardiopulmonary resuscitation accounts for many fractures of ribs and sternum. Use caution in opening the chest so as to preserve evidence of pneumothorax and air embolism. Air embolism is usually made obvious by distention of the heart and the presence of frothy fluid within the cardiac chambers and peripheral vessels. Record the quantity of fluid or blood within the pericardial sac and pleural cavities. Caution: Never discard fluid recovered from body cavities until after all known foreign objects or projectiles have been located.

Abdomen. Note the relationships of organs one to another. Measure any fluid present. Trace the course of injuries prior to removal of the organs. Preserve the gallbladder and urinary bladder intact to have the fluids available for toxicologic specimens if necessary. Remove the alimentary tract intact to prevent possible contamination of other viscera in case it is necessary to preserve organs for toxicologic examination. Attempt to locate projectiles prior to removal and dissection of organs.

Extremities. In all suspicious and all homicidal deaths, the hands should be protected from contamination by being covered with plastic bags.[4] The lateral surfaces of the arms, extensor surfaces of the forearms, and dorsal aspects of the wrists and hands should be examined in detail for evidence of defense wounds. Incised wounds of the palmar aspects of the hands and fingers are frequently seen in cases of stabbing. Observe each finger for evidence of broken fingernails or broken fingers. Trace evidence may be recovered from beneath fingernails; however, care should be taken not to inadvertently include tissue from the victim. The hands may be examined for powder residue employing neutron activation analysis or atomic absorption technics. Powder residue or blast injuries

---

[4] Editors note: Paper bags are sometimes preferable, particularly if the body is to be stored in cool temperatures. Less "sweating" or moisture condensation occurs.

may be noted on hands. Palmar aspects of hands and fingers may be examined by trace metal detection technics.

External genitalia. Examine for evidence of foreign material such as semen. Note any abrasions or contusions, their size, location, and number, and include evidence of injury along intertriginous surfaces of the thighs. To collect foreign hair samples use a fine comb to remove all loose hairs. Collect the hairs and place in identified containers. Aspirate fluid from vaginal canal for determination of acid phosphatase and blood group substance and examination for spermatozoa. Record obvious injury as possible source of hemorrhage.

Internal genitalia. Examine and describe the organs *in situ*. Remove carefully with blunt and sharp dissection using extreme care not to use instruments upon the cervix, which might confuse injuries produced by instrumentation on the cervix and uterus. Note and preserve any fluid or foreign material within cervix, uterus, or vagina.

Special Procedures

Collection of specimens. Have a variety of containers to meet individual requirements, such as, solid material, fluid material, and foreign objects. Collect tissue and fluids for chemical analysis in chemically clean containers. Identify each specimen as to organ or fluid. Label with the name of the deceased, the date, and the name of the examiner. Seal and store in the refrigerator or freezer. Hair samples may be obtained by plucking to secure entire hairs including roots. Obtain representative samples from several areas, and label each as to source, such as scalp or pubis. Take a sample of blood directly from the heart after opening the pericardial sac. A minimal sample is 100 ml. In cases of drowning take individual samples from both the right and left sides of the heart. Obtain all urine and bile that is available. Obtain adequate quantities of visceral organs and place each in a pint jar or equivalent container. Obtain samples from the stomach and small intestine, and identify individually. Preserve the chain of evidence by maintaining absolute control of specimens.

Observations relating to determination of the time of death include: (1) the stage of rigor mortis; (2) the degree, location, and fixation of postmortem lividity or livor mortis; (3) skin slippage, postmortem suggillations; (4) temperature of the body and viscera; (5) condition of the alimentary tract, the presence or absence of food, and the stage of digestion; (6) foreign items such as fly eggs or maggots; and (7) postmortem artifact or tissue destruction. These postmortem or putrefactive changes are secondary to the effect of scavenger insects and animals.

On the scene examinations may be helpful when possible to personally observe circumstances and conditions relating to the body.

Pitfalls that may be encountered include: the failure to make any of the preceding observations; the assumption of the cause of death and

5

failure to perform a complete autopsy; and the determination of time of death versus time of infliction of the fatal injury. An individual may sustain a fatal injury and survive for a long period of time prior to death.

Chapter II

FORENSIC AUTOPSY: A PROCEDURAL OUTLINE

Frank P. Cleveland, M.D.
Coroner, County of Hamilton
Cincinnati, Ohio

1. **Introduction, Concepts, and Principles**
    a. **Definition of medicolegal autopsy.** The medicolegal autopsy is difficult to define. Basically, it is an autopsy carried out under the laws of the State for the protection of its citizens. As such, the performance of the autopsy presupposes *State,* not *individual* permission. The importance to the State transcends the usual individual right to sepulcher until after the autopsy is completed.
    b. **Reasons for performing a medicolegal autopsy.**
        (1) To determine cause and manner of death.
        (2) To approximate time of death.
        (3) To identify, collect, and preserve physical evidence.
        (4) To provide factual information to law enforcement agencies, prosecutors, defense attorneys, families, news media and others with need to know.
        (5) To protect the innocent as well as to assist in the identification and prosecution of the guilty.
    c. **Requirements.**
        (1) Complete autopsy, no exceptions.
        (2) Thorough examination, overlook nothing.
        (3) Factual, objective written report without prejudice, advocacy, or theory.

2. **Preliminary steps.**
    a. Examine the body before removal of the clothing.
    b. Protect the clothing, body and hands from contamination; preserve clothing for examination at a later time.
    c. Note general state of the body.
    d. Observe the state of rigor and lividity.
    e. Determine the body temperature if applicable and other details as necessary to relate to the time of death.

3. **Autopsy procedures.**
    a. Note time and place of autopsy examination.

b. External examination: apparent age, height and weight, state of nutrition, scars, tattoos, color of eyes and hair, teeth, muscular development, abnormalities, deformities, and marks of hospitalization.

c. Detailed examination of injuries: size, shape, location, pattern, and relationship to anatomic landmarks.

d. Photographs.
   (1) To identify deceased.
   (2) To document injuries and their location (include scale for comparison).
   (3) To show relationship of external and internal injuries.
   (4) To demonstrate pathologic processes other than those of traumatic origin.

e. X-ray and fluoroscopic examination.
   (1) To locate bullets or other radiopaque objects.
   (2) To identify victim.
   (3) To document old fractures, recent fractures, anatomic deformities, metallic foreign bodies, plates, nails, and screws from surgical procedures, etc.

f. Internal examination.
   (1) General examination of head, neck, cervical spine, thorax, and abdomen.
   (2) Note course and direction of wound tracks within the body and in relationship to specific organs.
   (3) Note relationships and conditions of viscera.
   (4) Remember that antemortem and postmortem relationships of wounds and viscera may not always be the same.
   (5) Preserve evidence. Recover and identify foreign objects (bullets, fragments of knives, etc.); label and establish chain of custody.

g. Orderly examination of the body cavities and viscera.

4. **Procedures frequently used in forensic autopsies.**
   a. Collection of specimens.
      (1) Hair from scalp and pubis.
      (2) Comb pubic hair for foreign hairs.
      (3) Collect specimens of blood, urine, and bile.
      (4) Collect specimens of viscera, and body secretions.
      (5) Collect any likely material for examination to determine presence of semen and sperm.
      (6) Place specimens in chemically clean containers.
      (7) Store in refrigerator or freezer.
      (8) Properly identify and label specimens.
      (9) Preserve "chain of evidence"—control of specimens.
   b. Clothing.
      (1) Examine prior to removal.

    (2) Correlate defects with bodily injuries.

    (3) Remove and air dry if wet.

    (4) Label and preserve.

  c. Observations relating to estimation of time of death.

    (1) Rigor.

    (2) Lividity.

    (3) Temperature of viscera.

    (4) State of digestion of any food in the stomach.

    (5) Amount of urine in the bladder.

    (6) State of decomposition.

    (7) Fly eggs, fly larvae (maggots), and other insect activity present.

5. Postmortem artifacts.

  a. Artifacts of decomposition.

  b. Third party artifacts.

    (1) Animal activity: arthropophagy.

    (2) Insect activity: anthropophagy.

    (3) Emergency medical treatment in agonal and postmortem state.

    (4) Deliberate mutilation: dismemberment, etc.

  c. Artifacts of environment.

    (1) Postmortem burning.

    (2) Postmortem corrosion.

    (3) Postmortem maceration.

  d. Other artifacts.

    Artifacts of storage prior to examination.

6. Cautions.

  a. Do not fail to make any of the preceding observations.

  b. Do not assume the cause of death prior to actual completion of the autopsy.[1]

  c. Do not confuse time of death with time of inflication of fatal injury.

---

[1] Editors note: The autopsy is not over when the body leaves the autopsy room. At that point, toxicologic and histologic examination has just begun. Investigational data of great correlative importance may not yet be available to the prosecutor. Avoid premature dogmatic statements until all findings can be examined and correlated.

Chapter III
THE AUTOPSY PROTOCOL

John F. Burton, M.D.
Chief Medical Examiner of Oakland County
Pontiac, Michigan
and
Charles S. Petty, M.D.
Chief Medical Examiner, Dallas County
Director of Institute of Forensic Sciences
Dallas, Texas

Introduction

Narrative versus numerical form. A protocol is a signed document containing a written record which serves as proof of something. In pathology it is used in two basic forms: the narrative (in story form) and the numerical (by the numbers). Each form has its advantages and its disadvantages depending entirely upon the personal views and abilities of the individual prosecutor and his account of the autopsy findings; nonetheless, the end result using either form should be an accurate record of the autopsy findings.

1. **The narrative form**
   a. Advantages
      (1) For those of us who are very able at telling stories, the narrative protocol is balm to the reader and can be made poetic.
      (2) It provides an immediate storage of the facts on tape as it is dictated.
      (3) The pathologist is able to demonstrate, through narration, his personal attention and expertise by showing differences between normal and abnormal appearances.
   b. Disadvantages
      (1) The prosecutor can eventually be lulled into a repetitious form of dictation—"habit"—in which, except for summary of findings, all his protocols read alike and leave little room for individuality except for the final findings or diagnoses.
      (2) The narration of many pathologists is sketchy and sentence structure is incomplete with disconnected facts and descrip-

tion of immaterial data which in the finale reveals nothing informative. (Cross-examination of the pathologist on the witness stand regarding such a protocol is simply mayhem.)

(3) This type of protocol is not amenable to easy correction prior to typing the final or "smooth" copy.

(4) The narrative protocol tends to be both personal and subjective, neither of which are desirable features for courtroom purposes.

(5) It requires an expensive type of assistance: secretarial. There is a tendency for busy services to allow untranscribed protocols to collect and to become an unwieldy backlog.

2. The numerical protocol

a. Advantages

(1) It provides a guide for an orderly description of all autopsy findings and tends to prevent the omission of minor details, at times forgotten during narration.

(2) It provides a uniformity of detailed information on all cases.

(3) It facilitates immediate inspection of any particular heading, feature, or organic lesion found at autopsy.

(4) It is objective and impersonal, both desirable features in forensic practice.

(5) It is amenable to correction prior to final typing (if it is to be typed.)

b. Disadvantages

(1) Completion of the numerical protocol may require more time than the dictation of a narrative form.

(2) The format is not applicable to mummies, skeletons, unknown bones, four-footed animals and birds.

(3) If the numerical protocol is not typed, it may be difficult to read.

(4) It requires many pages, and therefore, more file space.

Examples of both the narrative and numerical form are to be found in the publication: Brinkhous, KM: Accident Pathology, Proceedings of an International Conference. US Government Printing Office, Washington, D.C., 1970, 249 pp. The interested reader is referred to this publication for a rather complete set of useful forms and body diagrams. These pages may be freely reproduced without obtaining specific permission; this was the intent of the editor and an objective of the conference which sparked the production of the book.

Preparation

Eventually and inevitably preparation of an autopsy protocol becomes a very personal matter. Availability of dictating equipment, habit, and even the geography of the autopsy area all enter into the production of the protocol. Many combinations of available personnel and equipment are in use to facilitate production of autopsy protocols.

1. Dictation in the autopsy room at time of autopsy.
   a. To a stenographer
   b. Using dictation equipment
2. Dictation after conclusion of the autopsy outside of the autopsy area.
   a. To a stenographer
   b. Into dictating equipment onto a permanent belt or disc.
   c. Into dictating equipment onto an erasable belt, disc, or tape (wire)
3. Write (longhand) or type protocol with own hands

Few pathologists will resort to (3) above. There are advantages and disadvantages to both (1) and (2). In the instances of an examination of a body with multiple external abnormalities, direct dictation at the time of examination is of great help in the production of an accurate, detailed report. A possible variation upon this procedure is to delay dictation of a very complicated external appearance until the photographs are available and then to describe the body relying upon the photographs and notes made at the time of the initial examination. There is some merit to this latter approach; the description of the body and its appearance as recorded by the camera will not vary.

Organization

The great advantages of delaying the actual dictation until after the autopsy is over, are the indisputed ones of organization, clarity, and avoidance of verbosity. It is much easier to organize thoughts, to express them clearly and to avoid "overspeak" when in the office, away from the bustle of the autopsy area and without interruption.

Each pathologist will undoubtedly develop his own particular method that will satisfy his requirements and those of his office. Local conditions will modify the "system" developed by any one individual.

In addition to the "system" of dictation, or recording of the data developed at the time of the autopsy, each pathologist will develop his own style and form of the autopsy record or protocol. His own language capabilities, his background, education, and experience, and the objectives of the autopsy in each instance, will modify any general scheme that might be adapted for use. The language, style, and organization cannot be detailed for all situations and for all prosecutors.

Some general guidelines for the organization of autopsy records may be mentioned:

1. External description
2. Evidence of injury
    a. External
    b. Internal
3. Systems and organs (cavities and organs)   Factual
4. Special dissections and examinations
5. Brain (and other organs) after fixation
6. Microscopic examination
7. Findings (diagnoses)   Factual and interpretative
8. Opinion (conclusion)   Interpretative and opinion
9. Signature

The usefulness of considering the "injury picture" in one or two sections of the autopsy report cannot be over-emphasized. Many medico-legal autopsies are performed because of true or suspected injuries caused by accident, a homicidal attack, or a suicidal effort. The core of the autopsy report is really the description of injury. To hide the details of the trauma among the general description of the organs is to deny the reader (who may not be a physician) the opportunity to see all of the injury described in one coherent paragraph. He must then search for individual fragments of the "injury picture" and try to synthesize from these bits and pieces of scattered information an overview of the entire injury pattern. This is a prolonged misuse of time. Why not make it an easy task?

A word about the findings. Traditionally, these have been labeled "diagnoses," but are they? In reality, the findings (and description) of a gunshot wound is much more a true finding than a diagnosis. So also is wet clothing in a death suspected to be due to drowning. Why not just label these as "findings"? If such is done, then includable are such combinations as:

1. Epilepsy
    a. History of seizure disorder
    b. Dilantin and phenobarbital found in blood
    c. No epileptogenic focus found

or

1. Drowning
    a. Found in lake
    b. Pulmonary edema (wet lungs)
    c. Maceration of skin of soles and palms
    d. Ingestion of water

Opinion

The opinion is the section of the autopsy report that the defense counsel and the insurance adjustor examine most closely. It should be phrased in simple, understandable English, avoiding medical terminology, and indicating the nature of the disease (injury) causing death and any major complicating factors. For example:

1. It is my opinion that Hazel Jaques, a 59-year-old woman, died of heart disease of the type occasioned by a gradual narrowing of the small arteries that supply the heart itself with blood. No injuries of significance were found at the time of autopsy.

2. It is my opinion that Martin Jewell, a 22-year-old man died as a result of a gunshot wound of the chest with the bullet passing through the left lung and heart and causing massive internal hemorrhage. A .38 caliber bullet was recovered. No evidence of close-range firing was noted. No other injuries or significant natural disease process was found at the time of the autopsy.

To fail to record an opinion is to fail to give a written synthesis of the central issues that caused the autopsy to be conducted. Such is an abrogation of the duty of the pathologist.

Corrections

There are two methods to effect correction of errors in the production of the final autopsy report or protocol. An effective method is to pencil in the needed correction and return the page to the typist for retyping. But what to do when the error is noted only after the record is signed, and copies have been released? An acceptable method is to draw a line through the word, phrase, or sentence it is desired to delete, write in the substituting word or words, and then initial the page in the margin opposite the correction. Needless to say, this should be done in ink, not pencil.

Certification

One of the duties of the medical examiner (or coroner) is to properly certify each death. Every State (or vital statistical registration area) provides forms designed for certification of death. Some registration areas provide special medicolegal death certificates especially designed for use by the medicolegal offices of that jurisdiction.

The pathologist to the coroner, or the pathologist, who performs only occasional medicolegal autopsies, may never have to actually complete the death certificate form. In other jurisdictions the pathologist is actually a deputy of the coroner and as such is empowered (and expected) to certify those deaths where he actually performs the autopsy or makes an external examination of the body. In other situations, the pathologist may serve in a less official manner to help complete the death certificate, or at least to advise the medicolegal officer of his opinion as to the cause and manner of death.

The following comments by one of us (J.F.B.) may be of use in day-

14

to-day solving of problems concerning death certification regardless of the precise role undertaken by the pathologist:

1. The certifier of death should give the cause and manner of death if he knows. If it is not known, the certificate should be signed out as "Pending." When the cause becomes known, he should sign an amended certificate giving the cause and manner of death.

2. The manner of death as requested on the death certificate falls within one of five categories: natural, suicide, homicide, accident, and undetermined. Such terms are already selected to classify the death of the subject and should not be transposed with diagnoses. For example, cause of death "pending," manner of death "pulmonary edema." On the contrary, if the cause of death is "pending," it follows that the manner of death is likewise "pending."

3. The cause of death should be given as the disease or condition that brought about the cessation of life. For example, a. gunshot wound of mouth, self-inflicted; manner of death: suicide; b. carbon monoxide asphyxia, house fire; manner of death: accident; c. shotgun wound of abdomen, manner of death: homicide; d. arteriosclerotic heart disease; manner of death: natural. Always keep the cause and manner of death distinctly separated.

4. The cause of death in medicolegal cases should be stated as briefly and concisely as possible with the idea in mind that at some future date you may be called to testify in court in regard to the death. It has been the experience of many, that usually such delayed hearings are exploratory from the legal standpoint and you will not be asked about the cause of death but about an insignificant finding instead. Do not volunteer irrelevant information on the death certificate. This can cause much trouble for many people including yourself. For example, a solitary occupant of an automobile was killed when his car was pinned in among ten other cars in a chain collision on an icy freeway. The pathologist signed the death certificate for the victim and indicated shock and hemorrhage due to multiple fractures and internal injuries as the cause of death. This would have been sufficient; however, in Part II of the death certificate (significant conditions not associated with primary cause of death) he listed bronchogenic carcinoma. This was based upon the discovery at autopsy of a small, solitary, noninfiltrative mass about 1 cm. in diameter, which was asymptomatic, and unknown to the man or his family. This small mass caused this pathologist and the family of the deceased agonizing days in court. His thoroughness was even criticized by the judge, since, if it was an incidental discovery and obviously not the cause of death, why was it on the certificate? One can make trouble for himself by being "too wordy" on a death certificate.

5. Finally, if after exhaustion of the means at your disposal, includ-

15

ing laboratory examinations and consultation, you are unable to arrive at a diagnosis with reasonable medical certainty, complete the certificate as "Cause of death: undetermined, manner of death: undetermined." This leaves the door open if future "clues" develop in the case. For example, some remorseful culprit may later confess to something that you had not dreamed was possible.

One available guide to medicolegal death certification is the U.S. Department of Health, Education and Welfare, Public Health Service, National Center for Health Statistics: *Medical Examiners' and Coroners' Handbook on Death and Fetal Death Registration,* published by the Government Printing Office, Washington, D.C., 1967.

Chapter IV
PRESERVATION OF MEDICOLEGAL EVIDENCE

Arthur J. McBay, Ph.D.
Chief Toxicologist
Office of the Chief Medical Examiner
Chapel Hill, North Carolina

Introduction

Evidence is legally acceptable to the courts only if it meets rigorous tests: (1) it must be obtained in a legal manner; (2) it must be relevant to the issue; (3) the chain of custody of the item must be intact and known; and (4) it must be evaluated by qualified expert examiners who are available to present their findings and their opinions concerning its interpretation or significance. The recognition, identification, and proper safeguarding of evidence is most important as there may be only one chance to procure it in a given case. Hence, the pathologist as well as the investigators should have plans for procuring and protecting evidence in all situations. This may require complete notes, photographs, x-rays, and proper containers, adequately labelled and identified.

At the Scene

Scenes of death may vary from a single room to an entire hotel, from an automobile in a remote area to a large airliner, and from an isolated and unpopulated area to a busy intersection in a large metropolitan city. As the medicolegal investigator frequently is not the first at the scene, the primary investigators must be educated not to alter anything which lies within the province of the medicolegal investigator. This requires that those responsible officials (*i.e.,* the local police or sheriff) who are most likely to be confronted with bodies and scenes of death, should be briefed ahead of time and specific arrangements should be formulated in advance for safeguarding the scene from "curiosity seekers" and "souvenir hunters."

The pathologist should have available a kit containing rubber gloves, a strong flashlight, syringes and needles, instruments (including forceps, scissors, surgical knife), labels, and containers for blood and organs. Plastic vials and jars are good for small samples such as hair, bullets, blood, and organs. Plastic bags are useful for organs, clothing and larger

17

articles, and to cover the hands[1] or other parts of the body. Larger plastic containers may be used for bodies. **No more than one article should be placed in a container.**

The medicolegal investigator first should observe the scene without disturbing anything and make complete notes describing everything. Notes should include not only what is observed but also things that are not present such as, no rings on fingers, no wallet or valuables in the pockets, etc. Specific notation that certain items (*e.g.,* the hands) have been examined may be useful.

The body may be described as well as its environment. Describe furniture, doors, windows, furnishings, stoves, weapons, blood and other stains and marks, medicines, drugs, glasses, and bottles. Temperature, weather, and other conditions should be noted. A complete set of photographs should be made. Usually the law enforcement agents will arrange this but the medicolegal investigator should be prepared to take pictures unless he is certain that others will. The scene should be examined by a fingerprint examiner followed by a trace evidence specialist. In addition to these specialists, the responsible law enforcement officers and the coroner, medical examiner, or his agents will examine the body. If the hands are to be examined for powder residue, blood, or other trace evidence, fingerprinting should be delayed and the hands protected by enclosing them in plastic bags[2] before removal from the scene. Agreement between law enforcement officers and the coroner or pathologist with respect to removal of clothing from the body should be reached in advance. As a general rule the clothing should be left intact on the body until additional photography is completed after removal of the body from the scene. If the clothing is removed prior to this it must be adequately described and removed without cutting or tearing. The clothing should be allowed to dry in warm air and then enclosed in properly labelled containers for transmission to the laboratory.

Any ligatures should be carefully photographed before removal, cut if necessary, leaving the knot or knots intact. The cut ends may be joined with string. Handling of weapons may destroy fingerprints and bloodstains as well as remove hairs, fibers, and other trace evidence. Therefore, objects should not be pushed into the wounds or defects in clothing. Firearms should be left in the condition they are found. If they are unloaded, the position of each bullet and casing should be noted. Bullets should be marked by an expert who will not alter the patterns used for identification. Finally, the body may be removed, preferably in a plastic bag, exercising care not to "manhandle" the body and possibly produce

---

[1] Editors note: Sweating may occur when the body is refrigerated prior to removal of plastic bags. Ordinary paper bags may cause less skin maceration.

[2] *Vidi supra.*

artifactual injuries, fractures, or otherwise damage the evidence still present on the victim.[3]

Opinions about wounds, trauma, cause and manner of death should be reserved until a detailed examination has been made or completion of the autopsy. In some cases the opinions should be delayed until after laboratory examinations are completed.

At the Autopsy

The means of identifying the body should be carefully recorded. The body should be photographed for identification and for overall appearance. The clothing, and any rings, or other jewelry should be described. The clothing should be removed without cutting or altering. If it is to be retained, it should be allowed to dry in air and should be properly identified. Then necessary x-rays should be taken. Any bullets or other foreign objects removed from the body should be placed into containers and labelled properly. Notes should be made identifying where the items were found to assist in future recall.

Blood and other specimens should be put into clean, dry labelled containers. The blood should contain 1 percent sodium fluoride as a preservative. The specimens should be refrigerated or frozen to preserve them. All specimens and items of evidence should be individually packaged. When the hands are to be examined, the bags[4] put on at the scene should be left intact until such time as specimens are to be procured.

The importance of establishing a written record—or receipt and release record—of evidence cannot be overestimated. We recommend evidence be transmitted in or attached to a form generally as follows:

Step 1	Step 2
Signature of Holder—Russell F. Fisher, M.D.	Sgt. J. W. Brown
Date—1/1/91	1/4/91
Item—.38 caliber bullet	.38 caliber bullet
Case Reference—Joe Doe—left chest	Joe Doe—left chest
Transferred to—Det. J. W. Brown	Crime Lab., City Police Department
Date—1/2/91	1/4/91
Signature of Recipient—Sgt. J. W. Brown	J. D. Smith

[3] Editors note: Obviously, teamwork among the medicolegal investigators, representatives of the law enforcement agencies, and the body movers, as well as other investigators (when the apparent nature of the death requires their presence) is the key to success. All have jobs to do, and each must avoid treading upon the toes of others. Failure to recognize and preserve evidence with actual destruction of evidence and chaos may result from a lack of integrated effort.

[4] Editors note: Sweating may occur when the body is refrigerated prior to removal of plastic bags. Ordinary paper bags may cause less skin maceration.

Additionally a signed receipt should be issued by Brown to Fisher when he receives the evidence and in turn by Smith to Brown etc. Alternately a photocopy of the envelope at each stage may be added to the file of the individuals transmitting the evidence.

Do's and Don'ts

1. Do prepare beforehand.
2. Do protect the scene.
3. Do allow wet clothing to dry.
4. Do identify all specimens.
5. Do provide information and adequate instructions in regard to specimens so as to assist and direct the chemist (or technician) in the examination and the evaluation of laboratory findings.
6. Do know to whom you give any evidence.
7. Do collect adequate samples.
8. Do store and transport specimens properly.
9. Do use clean containers.
10. Do take all medicinals and substances found on and about the body and at the scene.
11. Do evaluate all the evidence before making conclusions.
12. Do examine clothing before removing from the body; then remove and preserve any loose items.
13. Do have photographs prepared of the body and the scene.
14. Do not alter the scene needlessly.
15. Do not cut, tear, or otherwise alter clothing.
16. Do not put objects through defects in clothing or wounds.
17. Do not use instruments contaminated with embalming fluids to collect specimens.
18. Do not use cotton swabs to collect specimens of sperm.
19. Do not untie knots or cut material; make notes so that reassembly is possible.

Chapter V

POSTMORTEM CHEMISTRY OF BLOOD, CEREBROSPINAL FLUID, AND VITREOUS HUMOR

John I. Coe, M.D.
Medical Examiner, Hennepin County
Minneapolis, Minnesota

Introduction

Determination of postmortem chemistries may be of value in a variety of situations. Results obtained in such studies may demonstrate biochemical abnormalities responsible for death when no autopsy is performed, establish a cause of death when autopsy reveals no significant anatomic pathologic abnormality, help in the evaluation of the physiologic effects of recognizable anatomic lesions, and assist in estimating the time of death.

With the development of automation in the hospital laboratory, ease of performance and low cost makes routine examination of postmortem blood and body fluids practical. A sufficient body of published knowledge enables an investigator to interpret postmortem values for a wide variety of substances. It has been found that some biochemical materials in the blood remain remarkably stable after death while others show varying degrees of change. When changes occur they may or may not follow predictable patterns.

When marked changes from antemortem values have occurred in postmortem blood, other body fluids have been examined in an attempt to get a more accurate estimate of possible antemortem abnormalities. Cerebrospinal fluid was first studied and found to be of value for ascertaining certain abnormalities. However, collection of cerebrospinal fluid is inconvenient and often difficult to obtain free of blood and other contaminants. Further, changes in cerebrospinal fluid occur fairly rapidly and tend to be erratic. To obviate the problems associated with cerebrospinal fluid, there has been an increasing use of vitreous humor for chemical analyses. The eye is isolated and well protected anatomically so that vitreous humor is usually preserved despite serious trauma to the head and is much less subject to contamination or putrefactive change than either blood or cerebrospinal fluid. Most importantly it has been found that chemical changes for many substances occur much more slowly in vitreous humor than in the blood or cerebrospinal fluid. With

21

care, approximately 2 ml. of crystal clear fluid can be obtained from each eye. Material from one eye is sufficient for determination of electrolytes, urea nitrogen, and glucose, leaving material from the second eye for other constituents, duplicate analyses, or toxicologic procedures.

This chapter is an expansion of a review article[13] dealing with postmortem chemistry that was recently published by the author. It remains primarily a compendium of available data published in the English literature, regarding postmortem chemistry of blood, cerebrospinal fluid, and vitreous humor. Each type of fluid is discussed independently to provide the reader easy availability to general information and references for any particular substance in any of the fluids discussed. The use of the various fluids in evaluating pre-existing disease or in helping solve other forensic problems is discussed. A few comments are made regarding toxicologic analysis of vitreous humor.

The information provided here deals only with changes in the early postmortem period. This is defined as the interval between death and the onset of intravascular hemolysis rather than any particular number of hours. For individuals interested primarily in tissues, the book by Evans[24] on the chemistry of death is an excellent, although somewhat outdated, review of the biochemical changes observed in both the early and late postmortem periods.

Blood

Carbohydrates

Glucose. The first significant work with forensic application in the English literature was by Hamilton-Paterson and Johnson[34] in 1940. They demonstrated that glycolysis occurred in postmortem blood taken from peripheral vessels, while blood taken from the right atrium frequently had high glucose values from glycogenolysis. They further showed that extremital blood from diabetics had high levels of glucose and that glycolysis in such cadavers occurred much more slowly than usual.

Hill[36] in 1941, wrote a classic paper proving three significant points by animal experiments. First, he established that the elevated blood glucose usually found in the right atrium came from glycogenolysis in the liver; secondly, he established that glycolysis occurred at the same rate *in vitro* and *in vivo* approximately 12.8 mg/dl per hour); and thirdly, he proved that asphyxia would produce a noticeable increase in "terminal" blood sugar. Referring then to human postmortem studies he listed nondiabetic conditions associated with significant "terminal" elevations of glucose. These included carbon monoxide poisoning (values as high as 336 mg/dl), increased intracranial pressure (one example had 560 mg/dl glucose in postmortem extremital blood), and obstruction of the upper respiratory tract (in one instance of a death from hanging the postmortem glucose was 608 mg/dl). The peripheral hyperglycemia was never higher than 650 mg/dl in any condition other than diabetes.

Tonge and Wannan[89] in 1949, re-established that there were substances other than glucose which produced reactions in the tests usually performed and demonstrated that postmortem blood contained considerable quantities of nonfermentable reducing substances. They believe this accounts for the fact that by routine laboratory methods one almost never finds a zero value for "glucose" no matter from where a specimen is obtained or how long it is obtained after death. In contrast to Hill's experimental work, the rates of glycolysis *in vivo* and *in vitro* were found to be quite different so that appreciable levels of true glucose were detectable as long as 60 hours after death in some bodies in which the blood glucose was assumed to be normal at the time of death. Their paper includes on attempt at determination of glucose in a body with advanced putrefaction in which the level of reducing substances was over 2000 mlg/dl but true glucose was absent. Studying a wide variety of cases they substantiated Hill's observations of postmortem hyperglycemia in conditions other than diabetes. Elevated levels were found in two cases of hanging, two cases of acute coronary artery occlusion, one case with cerebral hemorrhage, and in one death due to electrocution. However, in none of these did the glucose level exceed 300 mg/dl. In studies of five deaths of diabetics only one value of glucose was less than 400 mg/dl.

Fekete and Kerenyi[25] in 1956, once more confirmed the marked variation between right and left ventricular serum glucose values and felt no postmortem "normal" could be established. Diabetics as a group had much higher blood glucose values but there was an overlap with samples from nondiabetic individuals. The most interesting finding was that newborns and infants less than 3 months of age had significantly higher postmortem glucose levels than normal adults (170.9 mg/dl compared to 96.8 mg/dl).

A more recent publication[71] offers nothing new.

Lactic acid. Jetter[41] studied 20 cases and found very small amounts of lactic acid were present normally in both plasma and erythrocytes during life (approximately 1 mEq/L). At 1 hour post mortem, the values were prominently increased (to about 20 mEq/L). There was a progressive increase so that 12 to 24 hours after death the lactic acid values were 50 to 75 times higher than normal antemortem concentrations.

Nitrogenous Compounds

Blood urea nitrogen. Sanders[73] in 1923, established the prolonged stability of urea in blood after it has been removed from the body. Paul[66] in 1925, first proved the stability of urea in the body by drawing samples from the same cadaver at varying intervals post mortem and showing that they remained constant in value from one-half hour after death until (in some instances) 2 days post mortem. This was true whether the urea nitrogen was within normal range or was markedly elevated.

Subsequent work by Pucher and Burd,[70] and Polayes and associates[68] and Naumann[57] suggested an increase in urea nitrogen after death. However, more recent work by Levonen and co-workers,[46] Jenkins,[39] Jensen,[40] Fekete and Kerenyi,[25] and Coe[14] have all established that concentrations of urea nitrogen in the serum postmortem closely approximate those in antemortem blood (shortly before death) irrespective of the procedure used (*i.e.,* urease or the carbomido-diacetyl method of Skeggs). This was found to be true for all concentrations of urea from normal individuals to those with severe uremia. Fekete and Kerenyi[25] found the level of urea nitrogen in postmortem blood from individuals who died suddenly to average 15.5 mg/dl. Coe[14] in a similar series found the average postmortem concentration to be 13.8 mg/dl. In contrast, Fekete and Kerenyi[25] found an average postmortem serum urea nitrogen of 47.4 mg/dl in blood from hospitalized patients who died without evidence of kidney disease. They felt, as does this author, that the apparent postmortem elevations of blood urea nitrogen reported by the earlier workers really represented agonal changes in hospitalized patients where the antemortem concentrations were frequently obtained several days prior to death.

Substantiating Paul's[66] earlier work, Levonen and associates[46] and Coe[14] have demonstrated how extremely stable urea is in the body post mortem. Coe found it to be the most stable of any substance studied and in the majority there were less than 2 mg/dl variation in specimens obtained over 100 hours apart from the same cadaver.

Creatinine. Sanders[73] in 1923, pointed out that creatinine, like urea, was remarkably stable in postmortem blood and remains constant in specimens stored for 2 weeks. Paul [66] found creatinine to remain stable in bodies from which two samples of blood were drawn at different postmortem intervals. This was substantiated by Polayes and colleagues,[68] Naumann,[57] Hamilton,[33] Jenkins[39] and Jensen.[40] The remarkable stability of creatinine in postmortem specimens was established best by Levonen and co-workers,[46] who found levels of creatinine increase an average of only 0.35 mg/dl in specimens taken 96 hours apart from the same cadaver. Several authors point out that creatinine levels are proportionately closer to known antemortem levels than urea nitrogen values from the same individual. Several authors point out that creatinine levels are proportionately closer to known antemortem levels than urea nitrogen values in specimens from the same individual. This is undoubtedly due in some cases to the fact that creatinine seems less apt to increase from those prerenal conditions causing an elevation in the serum urea at the time of death.

Nonprotein nitrogen. Sanders[73] demonstrated that the concentration of nonprotein nitrogen, in contrast to urea nitrogen and creatinine, increased in stored blood and that this increase could not be accounted for by an increase in ammonia and amino acids. Sanders' observations on stored blood were substantiated in specimens drawn from cadavers at varying postmortem intervals by Hamilton-Paterson and associates,[34] and by Schleyer.[75] When antemortem retention could be safely ruled out, Schleyer found that the increase in plasma nonprotein nitrogen values were predictable. Sufficiently so that values of less than 50 mg/dl could be expected to be derived from bodies dead for less than 12 hours.

Amino acid nitrogen. Pucher and Burd [70] demonstrated a sharp postmortem increase in concentration of the free amino acid nitrogen in the blood caused by enzymatic breakdown of proteins. This was further developed by Schleyer.[75] Values less than 14 mg/dl were usually found in intervals of less than 10 hours post mortem. Concentrations continued to increase (until enzymatic exhaustion). Values of more than 30 mg/dl were frequently found by 48 hours after death.

Ammonia. Schleyer[75] found, using Conway's method, concentrations of ammonia in plasma, taken from peripheral veins, to be in the 1 to 3 mg/dl range for several hours after death. There was a sharp rise after the initial 8-hour period.

Uric acid. Pucher and Burd [70] found an average concentration of uric acid to be 6.2 mg/dl in samples from ten individuals 8 hours post mortem. Naumann's[57] results were similar with an average serum value of 5.5 mg/dl in specimens obtained 6 hours after death.

Other Organic Compounds

Cholesterol and lipids. Naumann,[58] Enticknap,[21] and Glanville[31] have all demonstrated that the total serum cholesterol remains in the normal range after death. The average for Naumann's series was slightly above normal antemortem levels while Enticknap's was slightly lower. Glanville compared terminal antemortem and postmortem values in 26 patients and found very close correlation between the two. This was true at both high and low levels of serum cholesterol and with postmortem intervals extending over 90 hours.

In contrast to total cholesterol, Naumann[58] found the cholesterol esters to be markedly reduced by an esterase which remained active in postmortem blood. He felt that the level of cholesterol esters, as determined in the postmortem state, was not a reliable indicator of hepatic function.

Enticknap[21,22] showed other lipid substances such as total serum fatty acids, total lipoproteins, and beta lipoproteins were all remarkably stable post mortem with little reduction due to autolysis (one-half of 1 percent per hour or less).

Bilirubin. Naumann[58] found that postmortem bilirubin values were similar to antemortem values. However, this was based on a study of only 12 cases; the average total bilirubin for the group was 0.1 mg/dl higher than the upper limit of his established normal antemortem range. Coe[14] found in a study of 94 individuals with normal antemortem bilirubin levels that there was a small but definite increase in the average concen-

25

tration of bilirubin at increasingly longer postmortem intervals (0.2 mg/dl average increase in 2 hours; 0.7 mg/dl increase in 20 hours). However, in specimens from icteric individuals concentrations of bilirubin were nearly identical before and after death enabling one to determine the degree of antemortem jaundice from postmortem determinations.

Protein. Naumann[58] in 1956, reported the postmortem total protein and albumin/globulin ratios in specimens from normal individuals (determined by chemical means) was in the range found in antemortem specimens. Coe[11] showed there was no significant change between antemortem and postmortem values for total protein when determined by Auto-Analyzer using the biuret method. Albumin decreased an average of 4 percent.

Schlang and Davis[74] made the first detailed report of electrophoresis of postmortem sera. They demonstrated that the usual serum proteins were readily identifiable and that an increase in the beta globulins was a fairly constant finding. Robinson and Kellanberger[72] in 1962, presented a much more detailed study of paper electrophoretic analysis of antemortem and postmortem serum. In 20 cases they found that the overall shape of the postmortem patterns differed greatly from the antemortem in only two instances. Both manifested a high broad peak in the beta region. These peaks were believed to be due to hemolysis. Comparing all antemortem and postmortem specimens a decrease in the albumin, with unchanged alpha 1 and alpha 2 globulins, an increased beta globulin, and slightly increased gamma globulins, was found. The character of the increase in the gamma globulins was nonspecific and was not likely to be confused with a monoclonal peak found in patients with myeloma. Using a cellulose acetate matrix, Coe[11] compared antemortem and postmortem electrophoretic tracings obtained with specimens from 18 people and found good correlation except when there was hemolysis. In 16 cases with no hemolysis there was found to be a 4 percent decrease in albumin and a 5 percent increase in beta globulin. Other fractions remained essentially unchanged.

Both Brazinsky and Kellanberger[5] and McCormick[51] studied immunoglobulins and found good general correlation between antemortem and postmortem specimens.

Enzymes

Acid phosphatase. Enticknap[20] demonstrated that there was a marked postmortem elevation in acid phosphatase. Values more than 20 times the normal antemortem concentration were found by 48 hours after death.

Alkaline phosphatase. In 1956, Naumann[58] pointed out that alkaline phosphatase became elevated post mortem. He found an average concentration of 5.3 Bodansky units in 14 cases ten and one-half hours after death (normal antemortem range 1.5 to 4 Bodansky units). Enticknap[20] using the King-Armstrong procedure showed an increase in the alkaline phosphatase concentration through the first 48 hours post mortem. The average level at the end of 2 days was approximately 10 times the normal antemortem value. Coe's[14] work is in agreement (values doubled in 8 hours, tripled in 18 hours).

Amylase. Enticknap[20] demonstrated that amylase levels become elevated after death reaching the highest concentration on the second day with levels three to four times those found antemortem.

Transaminase. Hall [32] in 1958, reported a rapid, high postmortem rise of serum glutamic oxaloacetic transaminase in intracardiac blood but found little elevation in femoral blood from clinically well patients who died abruptly.

In contrast Enticknap[20] found a striking progressive postmortem increase in concentration of serum glutamic oxaloacetic transaminase in blood taken from blood vessels in the arm. The increase was roughly linear with time during the first 60 hours after death.

Lactic dehydrogenase. Enticknap[20] found a progressive postmortem increase in concentration of this enzyme which paralleled transaminase. The increase in concentration was roughly linear with time during the first 60 hours after death. From this a crude estimation of the postmortem interval was found to be possible.

Esterase including cholinesterase. Petty and associates[67] studied the true (erythrocyte) cholinesterase in 130 postmortem subjects and found an average 1.47 micromoles of acetylcholine utilized. There was no significant difference based on color, sex, age, or cause of death. The true cholinesterase remained stable. No significant difference was found between refrigerated and nonrefrigerated samples and no significant decrease in activity was noted in samples periodically analyzed up to 3 weeks after death.

Moraru and associates[53] reported on total cholinesterase (erythrocyte and pseudocholinesterase) using Fisher and Pope's colorimetric method. This was done with blood from 40 cases that was collected 10 hours to 3 days after death. They demonstrated that total cholinesterase was stable for 10 days in refrigerated samples but that the total cholinesterase found was subject to great individual variation. In deaths preceded by a long period of illness the concentrations of cholinesterase were found to be much lower (0.59 ± 0.26 micromoles/ml) when compared to concentrations in persons who died suddenly from trauma (1.34 ± 0.47 micromoles/ml).

Arnason and Bjarnason[3] in 1972, studied total serum esterase using starch gel electrophoresis with postmortem serums obtained between one-quarter hour and 30 days after death. Samples were taken from the same body at intervals. Six esterase fractions were demonstrated in sera taken from living individuals. Several fractions disappear in postmortem serum; one fraction becomes stronger, continuing to increase in strength for at least 100 hours after death; and at least one new fraction develops

27

that is not found in serum taken from live patients. The authors believe proteolytic enzymes are the cause of these changes.

Hormones

17-Hydroxycorticosteroids. Done and co-workers[19] studied 17-hydroxy-corticosteroids in blood samples obtained by intracardiac puncture from 64 individuals between 5 and 20 minutes after death. Levels frequently were found to be elevated; the highest values were found following acute illness (mean value 101 ug/dl). However, the levels found in a group of patients dying of fulminating encephalopathies (most often fatal craniocerebral trauma) in contrast, were lower with a mean postmortem plasma value of 21 ug/dl.

Cortisol. Finlayson[28] in 1965, established that postmortem concentrations of cortisol were the same as those during life and remained stable for at least 18 hours after death. In 15 infants cortisol values were found to vary from 9 to 29 ug/dl with an average of 17.7 ug/dl. Values found in specimens from 20 adults varied from 13 to 26 ug/dl with an average of 18.4 ug/dl. The results were similar when analyzing specimens obtained from the right atrium and the femoral vessels.

Adrenalin and noradrenalin. Lund[49] studied the postmortem catecholamines in the blood of normal individuals. He found the concentrations to be higher than the concentrations found in the blood of living patients with pheochromacytoma. These concentrations were as high as those found in samples of blood collected from cases of accidental fatal adrenalin poisoning. There was a significant difference in the adrenalin content of blood taken from victims of violent (27 ug/L) and natural (55 ug/L) sudden death. The difference was presumed to be due to a variation in the length of the agonal period. The lowest concentrations of adrenalin were found in those deaths which were most sudden.

Thyroxin and thyroid stimulating hormone. Coe[10] found T_2 values tend to decrease after death. The rate of decrease is individual and erratic. In some instances where no thyroid disease was present, the postmortem concentration was found to be in the range of that expected in hypothyroid individuals. In contrast TSH values showed only minor variations and remained in the normal range for 1 to 2 days after death.

Insulin. Postmortem insulin levels are under investigation by Sturner.[81] While he studied primarily concentrations found in bile,[88] he was also determining serum levels and in 25 cases he found serum concentrations to vary from 0 to 200 microunits/ml. In 22 of the 25 cases, insulin levels were under 100 microunits/ml. The three cases having values between 100 to 200 microunits/ml were diabetics who used exogenous insulin in treatment. All blood samples were obtained from the heart.

Lindquist[48] in 1972, demonstrated that postmortem serum insulin values are higher than those found in specimens from living, healthy individuals. He further found that in the same body there can be great variation in

28

concentration of insulin depending on the source of the serum. In 43 nondiabetic individuals dying from a variety of natural and traumatic conditions, concentrations of insulin in blood obtained from the right atrium averaged 187 microunits/ml (range 7 to 590) compared to 23 microunits/ml (range 5 to 55) in blood taken from the femoral vein. In one individual who died from an overdose of a tricyclic antidepressant, 2,400 microunits of insulin/ml of serum were found in the right atrium and 179 microunits/ml of serum obtained from the femoral vein.

Electrolytes

Sodium. The first direct reference in the English literature to sodium determinations in samples obtained post mortem is that of Jetter.[41] He found that serum sodium remained constant during the first 12 hours post mortem, then the level began to decrease. Several recent articles concerned with electrolyte changes after drowning have indirectly shown that the sodium values decrease post mortem. Coe[14] in a more detailed study has demonstrated that the sodium begins to decrease immediately after death, but that there is a great deal of individual variation in the rate of decrease. Least squares regression analysis of a large group of observations revealed the average rate of fall to be 0.9 mEq/L per hour.

Chloride. Jetter[41] reported that there was a decrease in plasma chloride due to an intracellular shift with an average concentration in the range of 80 to 90 mEq/L 24 hours after death. Schleyer[75] and other European workers have substantiated the plasma chloride decrease and report it to be at the rate of approximately 0.25 to 1 mEq/L per hour. In least squares regression analysis of a large series Coe[14] found the rate of fall to be 0.95 mEq/L.

Potassium. Jetter[41] pointed out that within 1 hour after death there was a marked increase in potassium levels. Values up to 18 mEq/L were found followed by an individual gradual increase in the levels. It has been shown by extensive work in blood banks and elsewhere[91] that the release of potassium from the cells occurs so rapidly after death as to make evaluation of potassium metabolism impossible.

Calcium. Jetter[41] states that calcium levels remain constant in the early postmortem period. Naumann[62] agrees. Jetter did not specify the method he used for determining calcium; it was probably the Clark and Collip procedure which was used by Naumann. This procedure is specific for calcium. In contrast magnesium interferes with the AutoAnalyzer procedure which uses cresolphthalein complexone. This results in an apparent rise in postmortem calcium levels.[8,14]

Phosphorus. Jetter[41] reported an increase of inorganic phosphorus in serum occurring as early as 1 hour post mortem and reaching levels of 20 mEq/L 18 hours after death. There was also an increase in organic phosphorus. This was substantiated by Schleyer.[75]

29

Magnesium. Jetter[41] pointed out that in the living individual the magnesium level in tissue is high in contrast to the level in plasma. He states that during the early postmortem period, tissue cell integrity seems to be maintained, so that there is only a mild increase in the magnesium level in plasma. When hemolysis occurs, however, plasma magnesium increases rapidly so that eventually levels of 20 to 30 mEq/L are found. Coe's[8,14] investigation of postmortem calcium levels using the cresolphthaline complexone method indicates that magnesium begins to leave the cell before significant hemolysis occurs giving a false elevation in calcium levels.

Carbon dioxide combining power and carbon dioxide content. Jetter[41] described a marked rapid decrease in the carbon dioxide combining power. He thought this probably was due to the postmortem production of lactic acid with immobilization of base as sodium lactate. Carbon dioxide content, however, remained constant. In contrast, Coe[14] found an apparent exponential decrease in carbon dioxide content which he felt was a technical artifact of the AutoAnalyzer procedure. The decline in serum values probably reflected the decrease in carbon dioxide combining power.

Blood Gases

Oxygen tension. In 1967, Mithoefer and colleagues[52] performed blood gas analyses using specimens from dogs in which fatal cardiac or respiratory arrest had been induced under controlled conditions. When the heart stopped before the breathing stopped, the pO_2 was greater than 25 mm Hg; when the reverse was true, the pO_2 was found to be less than 25 mm Hg.

Patrick[65] in 1969, reported his series of 28 deaths of children: 7 SIDS with a mean pO_2 of 13.7; 6 sudden "explained" deaths with a mean pO_2 of 21.0 and 15 random autopsy series with a mean pO_2 of 24.8 mm Hg. Included in the random autopsy group were cases where death had occurred 24 hours prior to sampling; in these oxygen tensions were found to be as high as 45 mm Hg.

Osterberg's[64] preliminary studies in 1973, support the conclusions of Mithoefer and associates.[52] Studies were made of accident victims with total brain death and normal heart action who were maintained on respirators. Determination of blood gases indicated pure asphyxial-type deaths when respirators were turned off while heart action was still normal. The same type of analysis revealed pure cardiac-type deaths in those patients who died in the coronary care unit with observed sudden myocardial arrythmias while receiving mechanical assistance with respiration. Results of postmortem arterial oxygen studies in the two groups are given in the following table:

OXYGEN TENSION—AORTIC BLOOD

| Cardiac arrest | | Respiratory arrest | |
P.M.I.*	pO$_2$	P.M.I.*	pO$_2$
1.5	53	1.5	12
2.5	73	2	8
2.8	82	3	6
6	70	4	7
9	35	6	10
11.8	40	9	3
22	44	15	3
		>15	3

* P.M.I. = postmortem interval in hours.

Cerebrospinal Fluid

Carbohydrates

Glucose. Hamilton-Paterson and Johnson[34] in 1940, first showed that the levels of glucose in cerebrospinal fluid were increased in hyperglycemic individuals. They demonstrated that glycolysis occurred, but progressed at a slower rate than in normal subjects. Naumann[57] in 1950, reported postmortem glucose values in cerebrospinal fluid. He considered cerebrospinal fluid glucose levels to be a much better indicator of diabetes than those levels resulting from analysis of peripheral blood. In nondiabetics the glucose in cerebrospinal fluid remained below 200 mg/dl. This was found to be true even in asphyxial deaths of the type found by Hill[36] that produce a terminal hyperglycemia. Values greater than 200 mg/dl, especially when acetone is found to be present were considered diagnostic of uncontrolled diabetes.

Fekete and Kerenyi[25] reported the amount of glucose in cerebrospinal fluid decreased very rapidly after death even when postmortem hyperglycemia existed. Cerebrospinal fluid values over 150 mg/dl were considered to signify antemortem hyperglycemia. Diabetics as a group had still higher postmortem sugar levels (average 212 mg/dl). They further make the statement that antemortem hypoglycemia cannot be recognized by determinations of sugar in cerebrospinal fluid post mortem.

Lactic acid. Schleyer[75] reports that the concentration of lactic acid in cerebrospinal fluid will increase after death. There is a sharp and fairly regular increase up to the tenth hour after death with a definite slowing of the increase and a great range of variability thereafter. These determinations were made with the hope that increases in lactic acid could be correlated with the postmortem interval; however, the expectations were not fulfilled.

Nitrogenous Compounds

Urea. Pucher and Burd[70] first reported urea levels in postmortem

31

cerebrospinal fluid. The average level of urea was 73 percent of that found in serum. Naumann[57] in 1949, reported cerebrospinal fluid levels of urea to be somewhat higher than normal antemortem blood levels. Nevertheless, Naumann considered the concentration in cerebrospinal fluid more closely reflected antemortem concentrations in serum than levels obtained from the analysis of postmortem blood. Jenkins[39] reported in 1952, that the postmortem levels of urea in cerebrospinal fluid were the same as, or somewhat lower than, the blood levels at death. He considered that the cerebrospinal fluid level could be taken as a reliable indicator of antemortem urea retention. Jensen[40] reported similar results and thought there was no overlap between values obtained from normal individuals (even with prerenal nitrogen retention) and from individuals with true clinical uremia. Fekete and Kerenyi[25] in 1965, reported that concentrations of urea in cerebrospinal fluid were constant for the first 36 hours after death, irrespective of the time of collection; the upper limit of the postmortem normal was found to be 25 to 30 mg/dl.

Nonprotein nitrogen. Hamilton-Paterson and Johnson[34] found that there is a progressive increase in nonprotein nitrogen with increasing time after death. This increase has been verified by Schleyer.[75] He demonstrated there was, in general, an arithmetic increase in the concentration during the first 30 hours post mortem, following which the rate of increase slowed. Values greater than 80 mg/dl found in the cisternal cerebrospinal fluid were of no use in evaluating the postmortem interval.

Creatinine. Pucher and Burd[70] found the 8-hour postmortem creatinine to average 1.6 mg/dl in cerebrospinal fluid taken in 10 instances. Bollinger and Carrodus[4] in 1938, demonstrated that concentrations of creatinine in cerebrospinal fluid reflected the blood concentrations and remained constant after death. This was substantiated by Naumann[57] and Jensen,[40] both of whom believed this was the best substance to analyze to evaluate kidney function. Naumann felt that mild degrees of prerenal uremia produced no significant increase in levels of creatinine.

Amino acid nitrogen. Pucher and Burd[70] in 1925, first described the postmortem increase in free amino acid nitrogen due to the enzymatic breakdown of proteins. This observation has been substantiated by several workers and most extensively studied by Schourup and Schleyer.[75] These investigators have demonstrated, in general, an arithmetic increase in values with longer intervals of time after death and considered the procedure to be of some use in estimating the postmortem interval for the first 20 hours after death.

Ammonia. Ozsvath is quoted by Schleyer[75] as having reported that generally there is a linear increase of ammonia in cerebrospinal fluid with increasing time after death. Concentrations of less than 1 mg/dl were found immediately after death but increased to over 8 mg/dl by 60 hours post mortem.

Uric acid and xanthine. Pucher and Burd[70] found uric acid levels in

32

cerebrospinal fluid to be 2.6 mg/dl. These determinations were made on 10 specimens obtained 8 hours post mortem. Average concentrations of uric acid on nine individuals increased from 1.7 to 2.6 mg/dl in 6 hours after death as reported by Naumann.[57] Praetorius[69] reported a 100-fold increase in xanthine and hypoxanthine after death. This was calculated from measurements of uric acid production. The initial concentration of xanthine and hypoxanthine was found to range from 0.25 to 1.50 ug/ml.

Creatine. Bollinger and Corrodus[4] demonstrated that in contrast to creatinine, creatine definitely increased in the cerebrospinal fluid following death. Naumann[57] found that concentrations increased progressively with increasing postmortem time. He did not attempt to use this as a method of estimating the postmortem interval. Schleyer[75] substantiated Naumann's work and believed it could be used to estimate the time between death and collection of the sample.

Other Organic Compounds

Urobilinogen. Naumann[55] demonstrated that urobilinogen will diffuse from blood to cerebrospinal fluid whenever the blood level is high and the cerebrospinal fluid-blood barrier is disturbed. There was a parallel between cerebrospinal fluid and urinary urobilinogen levels.

Bilirubin. Naumann[53] found in a study of 43 icteric individuals that total bilirubin was demonstrable in the cerebrospinal fluid by the method of Malloy and Evelyn. The ratio of bilirubin in the cerebrospinal fluid to that in the serum was 1:35. Direct acting bilirubin analyses were found to be in a cerebrospinal fluid to serum ratio of 1:45.

Transaminase. Dito[18] determined glutamic oxalacetic transaminase in cerebrospinal fluid on 73 cadavers at postmortem intervals varying from 2 to 70 hours. There was noted to be a progressive increase in enzymatic activity as the postmortem interval lengthened. However, an accurate estimate of the postmortem interval could not be made from a single determination because of the wide range of values obtained.

Electrolytes. Naumann[59] demonstrated that the concentration of many electrolytes changed significantly after death but not with a sufficiently close correlation with time to serve as a means of determining the postmortem interval. Values found for anions and cations in 131 cases where specimens were removed an average 10½ hours after death are compared to normal antemortem values as follows:

	Postmortem mEq/L	Antemortem mEq/L
Sodium	127.0	142.0
Chloride	113.0	125.0
Potassium	21.0	2.9
Bicarbonate	9.4	2.6
Calcium	2.4	2.5
Magnesium	2.9	2.0
Phosphorus	5.2	0.8

Potassium. Mason and colleagues[50] first noted the postmortem increase in cerebrospinal fluid potassium. They noted the concentration increased in proportion to the logarithm of the time interval for as long as 70 hours after death. Naumann[59] believed that the potassium increase was statistically predictable only; it could not be used for predicting time of death in an individual case. Fraschini and associates[29] also found increasing levels of potassium with increasing time after death and thought this might have forensic usefulness. Murray and Hordynsky[54] analyzed 46 specimens of postmortem cerebrospinal fluid. These specimens were obtained from persons dying in hospitals. They found that the average rate of potassium increase was constant in relation to time of death and to the temperature of the body. However, much individual variation is apparent in their graphs. Schleyer[75] later demonstrated that beyond the twentieth hour after death, estimates of the time of death are completely unreliable.

Vitreous Humor

In contrast to blood and cerebrospinal fluid, there are no normal "clinical values" for vitreous humor. Values presumed to be normal must be obtained from extrapolation of postmortem determinations, experimental studies using animals, and a few studies conducted on enucleated eyes. These latter studies are of questionable value because enucleation is never performed without disease or injury that may alter the levels of chemical constituents present. Although animal experiments can be carefully controlled, considerable variation in concentrations of chemical constituents have been demonstrated between different species. Therefore, conclusions derived from the studies frequently cannot be correlated with data obtained from analyses of postmortem specimens obtained from humans. For these reasons the subsequent sections will report only studies on human postmortem material. Reference to articles written in other than English will not be included.

Carbohydrates

Glucose. Naumann,[61] Sturner,[86] and Leahy[44] considered the normal vitreous glucose level to be approximately one-half that of serum and to be stable. However, in a study in which vitreous humor was obtained from the same individual at varying intervals after death, Coe[6] showed by the ferricyanide reduction method that the initial levels were approximately 85 percent that of the serum. Subsequent study[12] revealed that when a glucose oxidase procedure is used, rather than ferricyanide reduction technic, lower absolute values and a lower ratio of vitreous humor to serum values are obtained.

Coe[6] demonstrated there is a consistent decrease in levels of vitreous humor glucose in nondiabetic individuals with increasing postmortem interval. The postmortem decrease could be great and very precipitous decrease was noted in some instances. Very low concentrations of glucose in vitreous humor, considered by Sturner to be indicative of hypoglycemia (25 mg/dl), were shown to be a result of postmortem change. Coe[6,12] felt it impossible to make a diagnosis of hypoglycemia except in a very few circumstances. All authors have found, however, that the determination of vitreous humor glucose level is a valuable tool for diagnosing antemortem hyperglycemia. This, when used in conjunction with a test for the presence of ketone bodies in the vitreous humor, is useful to determine diabetic acidosis.

Lactic acid. Jaffe[38] found the concentration of lactic acid increased after death from an initial value of 80 to 160 mg/dl to 210 to 260 mg/dl after 20 hours.

Pyruvic acid. Jaffe[38] reported that the concentration of pyruvic acid decreased rapidly after death from 2 to 3 mg/dl to 0.1 to 0.2 mg/dl after 10 hours.

Ascorbic acid. Jaffe[38] found vitreous humor contained the highest concentration of ascorbic acid in the body. The levels decreased slowly within the first 20 hours. The initial concentrations obtained during the first hour post mortem range from 19 to 38 mg/dl. Gantner and co-workers[30] studied materials in 32 cases. They found the baseline levels to be extremely variable ranging from 2.0 to 22.0 mg/dl. Analysis of sequentially obtained samples showed a tendency for the concentration of ascorbic acid to increase during the first 5 hours after which the values slowly decreased.

Nitrogenous Compounds

Urea. Naumann[61] considered the postmortem urea level in the vitreous humor to be moderately elevated. His study, however, was performed using hospitalized patients whose blood urea nitrogen levels were probably above normal at the time of death. In contrast to Naumann's work, Leahy and Farber[44] found the vitreous humor urea level to be within the normal range for individuals who die suddenly. Also, the vitreous humor level of urea was found to be normal in those persons in whom the blood urea nitrogen level was known to be normal just before death. Coe[6] found the vitreous humor urea nitrogen paralleled the blood urea nitrogen over all ranges of urea retention. Further, it was by far the most stable of all vitreous humor constituents studied in the postmortem state. In more than 90 percent of the cases there was a variation of less than 3 mg/dl between specimens drawn over 100 hours apart.

Creatinine. Naumann[61] found vitreous humor creatinine levels to be normal after death as did Leahy and Farber.[44] All of these investigators found the levels in vitreous humor to be slightly lower than serum creatinine levels. Naumann found an average postmortem vitreous humor creatinine level of 1.2 mg/dl compared to average serum creatinine levels of 1.5 mg/dl from the same individuals. In five individuals with terminally elevated blood and vitreous humor urea nitrogen levels, Leahy and Farber found that the vitreous humor creatinines remained at normal levels.

Nonprotein nitrogen. Jaffe[38] in a study of 13 cases found the concentrations of nonprotein nitrogen increased erratically after death with no consistent pattern detectable.

Uric acid. Sturner and colleagues[85] investigated vitreous humor uric acid concentrations in 44 individuals who died from a variety of traumatic causes and natural disease processes, among whom normal levels of uric acid in serum would be expected. Values for uric acid in vitreous humor varied from 0.7 to 3.0 mg/dl. In those 22 cases where the average postmortem interval was 4 hours, the average uric acid level was 1.3 mg/dl, but in the remaining 22 individuals where the average postmortem interval was 16.5 hours, the average uric acid level was 1.5 mg/dl.

Other Organic Compounds

Enzymes. Leahy and Farber[44] analyzed vitreous humor for lactic dehydrogenase, glutamic oxalic transaminase and glutamic pyruvic transaminase. When any activity was noted it was minimal. There was no apparent correlation with either normal or elevated antemortem concentrations of these enzymes in serum. Coe[6] found values of vitreous humor glutamic oxalic transaminase varied markedly with values ranging from 12 to 205 units. The values had no apparent relation to antemortem blood values or to any pathologic condition in the eye or elsewhere in the body.

Proteins and amino acids. The concentration of soluble protein in vitreous humor in man is 40 to 80 mg/dl. Vilstrup and Kornerup[90] using paper electrophoresis found the protein in a purified sample of human vitreous body to be composed of albumin and globulin in a ratio of 46:54. Normal human serum had a ratio of 74:26. Cooper, Halbert, and Manski[16] demonstrated by immunochemical analysis of the vitreous humor that a large number of serum proteins were present. They found one protein in the alpha globulin fraction in concentrations higher than in the serum which suggested to them a possible selectivity on the part of the human vitreous humor. Human vitreous humor was also found to contain a number of antigens not seen in serum; the origin, chemical composition, and localization of these were not determined. Finally, Erdei and Vass[23] demonstrated the presence of free amino acids in the vitreous humor by paper chromatography and found them to be identical to amino acids liberated from the vitreous humor by the enzymatic action of elastase. It was their tentative conclusion that autolysis due to proteolytic enzymes was responsible for the presence of these free amino acids in the vitreous body.

Bilirubin. Coe[6] found no evidence of bilirubin in the vitreous humor when using the Jendrassik and Grof procedure, even in individuals with jaundice. However, Naumann and Young[63] using the classic Malloy and Evelyn method found that bilirubin does enter the vitreous humor in small amounts. In 43 icteric individuals with an average serum concentration of 8.6 mg/dl, the vitreous humor contained bilirubin in amounts of 0 to 0.48 mg/dl with an average of 0.04 mg/dl. This gave a vitreous humor to serum ratio of 1:220 for total bilirubin while the ratio for direct acting bilirubin was 1:480.

Electrolytes

Sodium. Naumann[61] found vitreous humor sodium values to vary from 118 to 154 mEq/L with an average of 144 mEq/L. Leahy and Farber[44] in a smaller series found a range of 128 to 158 mEq/L and substantiated the postmortem instability of this substance. In two patients with antemortem hypernatremia they found the concentration of sodium in vitreous humor to be significantly elevated. Coe[6] similarly found sodium was extremely stable in the early postmortem interval. There was a much narrower range of normal values determined in 145 individuals where values were found to vary from 135 to 151 mEq/L with an average of 143 mEq/L. Coe[6] in studying hospitalized patients with both hyponatremia and hypernatremia found that vitreous humor values greater than 155 mEq/L or less than 130 mEq/L paralleled deviations in serum values which had been found to exist prior to death.

Chloride. Naumann[61] found an average vitreous humor chloride of 114 mEq/L. Leahy and Farber[44] reported that the range in normal individuals varied from 108 to 142 mEq/L. Thirty-nine patients with normal antemortem serum chloride values were examined. Coe[6] found chlorides to range from 104 to 132 mEq/L with an average of 120 mEq/L. As was true with sodium the vitreous humor concentrations remained almost constant for an average of 18 hours post mortem. Sturner and Dempsey[84] reporting on vitreous humor values found in 44 infants, who died suddenly and unexpectedly, an average of 120 mEq/L. Chlorides below 105 mEq/L or over 135 mEq/L, therefore, probably indicate antemortem hypochloremia and hyperchloremia.

Carbon dioxide content. Coe[6] found the carbon dioxide content as measured by the Autoanalyzer to vary from 4 to 26 mEq/L with an average value of 15 mEq/L. This was surprisingly stable showing a decrease of only 2 mEq/L in 15½ hours.

Calcium. Naumann[61] found an average concentration of 7.2 mg/dl in his series of 211 cases with an average postmortem interval of 9 hours. Coe[6] found concentrations of calcium to remain constant during the early postmortem interval and vary from 6.0 to 8.4 mg/dl with an average of 6.8 mg/dl. Coe found by studying several hospitalized patients with terminal hypocalcemia that the vitreous humor calcium was within normal limits. Sturner[85] also reported a similar range of normal values

37

for vitreous humor calcium. He also noted a lower concentration of calcium in several traumatic deaths for which no explanation was apparent.

Magnesium. There has been no extensive investigation of vitreous humor magnesium. The only report available is that of Sturner[80] who found a range of 1.5 to 2.5 mEq/L of magnesium in a series of 24 adults. Concentrations of 2.0 to 3.9 mEq/L, determined by atomic absorption spectrometry, were noted in a series of 20 infant deaths. The causes of death and postmortem intervals in these cases were not noted.

Phosphorus. Naumann[61] reported the concentration of inorganic phosphorus to vary from 0.1 to 3.3 mEq/L with an average concentration of 1.2 mEq/L.

Iodine. DeJorge and Jose[17] found the vitreous humor iodine in five postmortem enucleated adult normal eyes to vary from 5.1 to 5.9 ug/100 grams of fresh tissue with an average value of 5.44 ug/100 grams.

Potassium. Jaffe[38] first noted that potassium levels increased in the vitreous humor as the interval from death to sampling increased. This was later substantiated by Adelson and associates,[1] Hanson and colleagues,[35] Hughes,[37] Lie,[47] Sturner,[77] Sturner and Gantner,[87] and Coe.[6] Adelson established that the rise was arithmetic for any group and independent of environmental factors. The average rate of increase was 0.17 mEq/hour. Other investigators substantiated Adelson's work, but there was variation in the degree of correlation between the concentration of vitreous humor potassium and the postmortem interval. Sturner and Lie both found such close correlation that they believed the method could be used to predict time of death with a confidence limit of ± 5 hours. Adelson, Hughes, Hanson, and Coe all found such individual variation that the confidence limit of the method exceed ± 10 hours during the first day after death. Hanson and associates and Coe further showed that the standard error continued to increase as the postmortem interval increased. Most recently Adjutantis and Coutselinis[2] have attempted to improve the accuracy of predicting the postmortem interval by collecting specimens of vitreous humor from each eye at different postmortem intervals and by plotting the slope back to a theoretical "normal" value of 3.4 mEq/L. They felt that this method is satisfactory only during the first 12 hours after death, but this technic enabled them to estimate the time of death within ± 1.1 hours.

Osmolality. Sturner and associates[85] determined the osmolality of the vitreous humor in 45 cases and estimated the range for osmolality in all cases to be from 280 to 350 mOsm/Kg. The osmolality was noted to be increased proportionately to the concentration of ethyl alcohol present in the blood. In those cases with no alcohol present the normal range (including two standard deviations) was 288 to 323 mOsm/Kg with an average of 305.7 mOsm/Kg.

Toxicology. While toxicologic procedures would not normally be considered as part of a discussion of postmortem chemistries, there is a small body of knowledge indicating the usefulness of the analysis of vitreous humor for toxic substances. This may be of particular value when analysis of other body fluids is impossible or undesirable.

Alcohol. Four papers[15,26,45,83] have been published regarding determination of alcohol in the vitreous humor. These indicate that specimens of vitreous humor are satisfactory for determination of alcohol by any of the procedures now in common use (dichromate reduction, gas chromatography, alcohol dehydrogenase). There is some discrepancy between the reports as to the ratio of blood to vitreous humor alcohol. However, Coe[15] in the largest published series obtained a factor of 0.89, *i.e.,* blood alcohol equals 0.89 times vitreous humor alcohol. Scott[76] demonstrated that determination of alcohol using vitreous humor even after embalming gave reliable information regarding concentrations found in the vitreous humor prior to the embalming procedure. This is true if the embalming fluid contains no ethyl alcohol and the procedure used for the determination is specific for ethanol.

Barbiturates. Felby and co-workers[27] in a study of 19 individuals demonstrated that barbiturates were found in vitreous humor after diffusion equilibrium in concentrations equivalent to an ultrafiltrate of the blood. Coe[12] in a study of more than 17 cases of barbiturate poisoning substantiated that barbiturates enter the vitreous humor. He did not find as good a correlation between serum and vitreous humor as reported by Felby and colleagues.

Other compounds. Felby and co-workers[27] and Coe[12] found there was diffusion of meprobamate into the vitreous humor. Sturner[81] has found propoxyphene and pentazocine in the vitreous humor in concentrations approximately 25 percent of those found in the serum. Other drugs such as amitriptyline and digoxin have also been demonstrated to diffuse into the vitreous humor. Coe[12] has found ethchlorvinyl in the vitreous humor. In three cases of salicylate poisoning he found vitreous humor levels greater than 60 percent of the serum levels.

Discussion

Studies of glucose and insulin concentration and oxygen tension in blood samples obtained in the postmortem state, all demonstrate very significant differences in specimens taken from the right side of the heart and those obtained from peripheral blood vessels. When more sophisticated studies of blood components such as hormones, gases, and enzymes are performed, it will undoubtedly be most important to accurately identify the source of the material examined. Blood obtained by blind cardiac puncture or pooled mixed blood from the heart will not be satisfactory for analysis. The author for several years has used only specimens obtained from peripheral vessels. If the body is not to be examined internally, subclavian puncture is almost invariably productive of a sufficient sample of blood for analysis. A variety of peripheral vessels are available to the prosector when an autopsy is performed. Such specimens most closely resemble the blood that is routinely obtained from the living individual and are thus the most logical for comparison with antemortem constituents.

When vitreous humor is obtained specimens should be collected slowly with a syringe and a 20 gauge needle rather than with a vacuum tube and needle. The strong negative pressure of the latter frequently detaches fragments of the retina and contaminates the specimen. Tissue fragments (or blood) will alter analytical results significantly. Only crystal-clear colorless vitreous humor should be used. It is also important that all the easily aspirated fluid be withdrawn from the eye. That this is important is established by experimental facts: in the putrefactive phase electrolytes and other solutes vary in concentration within different areas of the vitreous body until diffusion equilibrium has been reached. This unfortunately precludes serial sampling from a single eye to determine gradients of postmortem change.

With proper specimens for examination, coordination of data presented for each fluid individually can show how postmortem chemistries may best be utilized to elucidate a number of clinical abnormalities.

Postmortem levels of glucose in blood are subject to such vagaries as to make evaluation of carboyhdrate metabolism difficult. However, antemortem diabetic hyperglycemia may be diagnosed from postmortem serum values when it is known that the blood examined is from a peripheral vessel, the postmortem interval is short, the deceased did not die from any condition that may produce a terminal elevation in glucose, and finally, that the values exceed 500 mg/dl. Confidence in the significance of the serum glucose level will be increased by the demonstration of glucose in the urine and/or the demonstration of ketone bodies in the blood or other body fluids.[42]

Because of the difficulties in interpreting levels of serum glucose in specimens obtained after death many investigators believe a diagnosis of antemortem hyperglycemia is made with greater confidence by examination of cerebrospinal fluid[25,26] or vitreous humor.[7,9,86] Of these two, vitreous humor is the easiest obtained and the least apt to change from terminal conditions that produce marked elevation in levels of serum glucose. Values over 200 mg/dl were never found in the vitreous humor by this author without an antemortem hyperglycemia due to diabetes or some other cause. Diabetic acidosis was easily diagnosed by demonstrating ketone bodies in the vitreous humor.

Unfortunately, extensive work on blood, cerebrospinal fluid, and vitreous humor have demonstrated that glycolysis occurs in each of these substances after death, and work of this author[6] reveals that glycolysis in

40

the vitreous humor may be precipitous. As a consequence it seems impossible in the light of our current knowledge to diagnose antemortem hypoglycemia with any degree of assurance as has been pointed out by both Coe[6,9,12] and Naumann.[60] Hypoglycemia may be considered likely when some predisposing condition such as starvation, chronic alcoholism with severe fatty metamorphosis of the liver, or an islet cell tumor of the pancreas is found in conjunction with values of glucose less than 20 mg/dl by ferricyanide reduction in specimens of vitreous humor obtained less than 3 hours after death.

In contrast to difficulty in evaluating carbohydrate metabolism, evidence of nitrogen retention is easily obtained from examination of any of the fluids discussed. It has been unequivocally established that in postmortem serum, cerebrospinal fluid, and vitreous humor obtained after death, the levels of both urea nitrogen and creatinine accurately reflect the terminal antemortem levels in blood. Further, there has been found to be great stability of these substances through the entire prehemolytic interval. A number of authors[7,9,12,33,40,44,46,56] have discussed utilization of urea and creatine levels in specimens obtained after death to evaluate the degree of renal disease and to establish uremia as the cause of death when no medical history or postmortem examination is possible. The author[9,12] has used mild degree of urea retention combined with hypernatremia to diagnose dehydration.

In contrast to urea nitrogen, there is a gradual increase in the level of nonprotein nitrogen which makes it unsuitable for evaluation of antemortem nitrogen retention.

The inability to evaluate antemortem abnormalities of electrolytes by examination of specimens obtained after death has been a problem for pathologists. This is still a problem when attempting to evaluate potassium metabolism and blood pH. However, recent studies of the vitreous humor have demonstrated that marked abnormalities in serum sodium and chloride will be reflected in abnormal vitreous humor values and further that the levels in vitreous humor remain constant for prolonged postmortem intervals. As a result, Coe[7,9,12] has found it possible to demonstrate the presence of antemortem hypernatremia and hyperchloremia in cases of neglected children and incapacitated adults.[7,9] Decreased levels of both sodium and chloride have been demonstrated in some infants dying with the findings of the sudden infant death syndrome,[12,84] in the presence of pyloric obstruction with prolonged vomiting[7,9] and in some alcoholic patients dying suddenly with no apparent pathologic abnormalities other than fatty metamorphosis of the liver.[82]

Study of a large number of cases involving abnormalities of electrolytes and urea reveals four common patterns to exist.[12] These are as follows:

(1) Dehydration pattern. This is characterized by simultaneous elevation of levels in the vitreous humor of sodium (over 155 mEq/L),

41

chloride (over 135 mEq/L) and moderate elevation of urea nitrogen (usually 40 to 100 mg/dl).

(2) Uremia pattern. This differs from the dehydration pattern in that there are marked elevations of urea and creatinine levels in vitreous humor and serum without significant increases in values for sodium and chloride.

(3) Alcoholic liver pattern. Characteristically this has a low concentration of vitreous humor sodium (less than 130 mEq/L), chloride (less than 105 mEq/L), and relatively low potassium (less than 15 mEq/L). Concomitant serum values will frequently reveal some elevation of bilirubin and occasionally values for urea nitrogen will be below 5 mg/dl.

(4) Decomposition pattern. Like the alcoholic liver pattern, there is a low concentration in the vitreous humor of sodium and chloride. However, there is a high vitreous humor potassium level (over 15 mEq/L) indicating a long postmortem interval.

It has long been known that calcium remains constant in the serum during the early postmortem interval. However, there is no literature available to indicate that any antemortem abnormalities of calcium metabolism have been ever diagnosed after death. Further work is necessary to prove that clinical cases of hypocalcemia and hypercalcemia can be diagnosed by an examination of the calcium in specimens obtained after death. However, as discussed earlier, this will not be possible with the Autoanalyzer utilizing the cresolphthaline complexone method.

Total cholesterol and other lipid substances in the serum have been shown to be stable after death. Some successful correlations of the presence of heart disease with abnormalities of fatty constituents of the blood [21,22,78] have been made. The stability of cholesterol also means that postmortem evaluation of the total serum cholesterol can be used to evaluate liver function and thyroid dysfunction.

It has been demonstrated that the values of serum bilirubin in samples obtained after death accurately reflect the antemortem degree of jaundice. The author[14] has demonstrated an apparent slight rise in postmortem values of bilirubin. This makes determination of the bilirubin level unsatisfactory for the evaluation of minimal chemical jaundice in equivocal cases of hepatic disease. Determination of proteins in specimens obtained after death accurately reflect antemortem values and inversion of the albumin/globulin ratio has the same significance as it does before death. All enzyme determinations used to demonstrate hepatic disease are of no value after death. This is because of erratic behavior which makes their values uninterpretable.

Determination of postmortem serum proteins by chemical analysis, electrophoresis, and immunoelectrophoresis reveals that they accurately reflect antemortem levels of the various fractions. Such determinations have been extensively employed[11] to demonstrate that no hypogammaglobulinemia exists in the majority of instances of sudden infant death syndrome. The author has demonstrated true agammaglobulinemia in a postmortem blood specimen collected from an individual known to have this condition prior to death. He has further demonstrated monoclonal elevation of gammaglobulin in serum obtained after death from an individual who died of myeloma.

Many studies have shown that variations occur quite rapidly in most enzymes (acid phosphatase, alkaline phosphatase, amylase, transaminase, lactic dehydrogenase, etc.) after death. Some of these variations are accompanied by changes in the physical characteristics of the enzymes themselves.[3] Certain physical properties of serum obtained after death vary from those collected prior to death.[20,43] In contrast to these enzymes, both true and total blood cholinesterase activities are stable for prolonged periods after death. Therefore this is of great significance to the forensic pathologist who may establish exposure to organic phosphorus poisons by the decrease in blood cholinesterase values.[67]

Study of postmortem levels of hormones is just beginning. The limited data available have already indicated that in cases of Waterhouse-Friderichsen syndrome there may be normal levels of cortisol in the blood after death. The author has found a postmortem cortisol level an aid in excluding Addison's disease as a cause of death in an individual who died with hypoplastic adrenal glands. Thyroid function studies done on blood specimens obtained after death have also helped the author to evaluate severe chronic thyroiditis found at autopsy.[10] Finally, knowledge of postmortem values for insulin has enabled both Sturner[88] and the author to diagnose cases of insulin poisoning.

Study of blood gases after death has received little attention to date. Experimental work indicates that asphyxial deaths may be distinguished from cardiac arrhythmias by the determination of oxygen tension in blood obtained after death from the left ventricle. This receives support from Osterberg's preliminary studies.[64] Patrick[65] believed the low oxygen tension found in babies dying of sudden infant death syndrome was an indication that the deaths were associated with respiratory obstruction or cessation of respiration before cardiac action ceased.

Coe[15] has found the alcohol level in vitreous humor to support the serum value when there is a question of possible contamination of blood specimens by tissue or other body fluids in instances of severe trauma. More recently, Scott[76] has demonstrated that vitreous humor collected from an embalmed body can be used to determine the presence of alcohol when no blood was available for analysis. The results quite accurately reflect the value that would have been found in the body prior to embalming. The establishment of the fact that a number of toxic substances do diffuse into the vitreous humor[12,27,79] will undoubtedly become of increasingly greater value.

Concerning the usefulness of chemical analyses in the determination of the postmortem interval: Schleyer[75] in his excellent review article has evaluated the chemical determinations in serum and cerebrospinal fluid and he found that tests for amino nitrogen, nonprotein nitrogen, creatinine, ammonia, and inorganic phosphorus, have some prognostic value. However, the range of error for each individual test is great. Therefore, for greatest accuracy, combinations of chemical determinations must be obtained as listed below (taken from Schleyer's review):

	Time since death (hr.)	
	Maximum	*Minimum*
Amino nitrogen		
Not exceeding 14 mg/dl (plasma and cisternal fluid) ..	10	
Non-protein nitrogen		
Not exceeding 50 mg/dl (plasma)	12	
Not exceeding 70–80 mg/dl (cisternal fluid)	24	
Creatine		
Not exceeding 5 mg/dl (plasma and cisternal fluid) ...	10	
Not exceeding 10 mg/dl (cisternal fluid)	30	
Not exceeding 11 mg/dl (plasma)	28	
Ammonia		
Not exceeding 3 mg/dl (plasma)	8	
Not exceeding 2 mg/dl (cisternal fluid)	10	
Inorganic phosphorus		
Exceeding 15 mg/dl (plasma and cisternal fluid)		10

The author prefers the use of vitreous humor potassium levels to the tests suggested by Schleyer. In temperate climates, potassium diffuses slowly into the vitreous humor. Therefore, potassium levels can be used as a measure of the postmortem interval over a longer period of time than can any of the substances so far studied in blood or cerebrospinal fluid. This is shown in Figure 1 taken from some of the author's previously published work. The accuracy of estimating the postmortem interval using a single vitreous humor potassium determination is subject to great error.[12] However, this would appear to be at least as reliable as any of the other chemical tests so far developed. Possibly drawing fluid from each eye at different times as suggested by Adjutantis and Coutselinis[2] will increase the accuracy of the method even when the procedure is carried beyond the 12 hours limit as recommended by the authors.

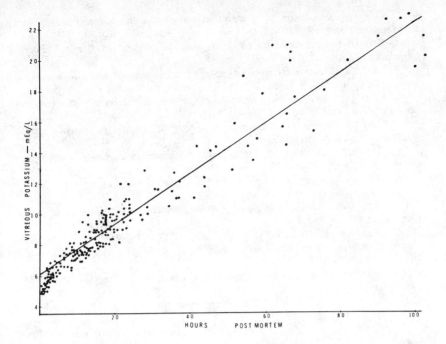

Vitreous potassium values of normal individuals plotted against the time after death with the line of least squares regression for all values having a postmortem interval of more than 6 hr. The slope is 0.1625 mEq. per hr. and the intercept is 6.19 mEq. per l.

References

1. Adelson, L, Sunshine, I, Rushforth, NB, et al: Vitreous potassium concentration as an indicator of the postmortem interval. J Forensic Sci 8:503–514, 1963

2. Adjutantis, G, Coutselinis, A: Estimation of the time of death by potassium levels in the vitreous humor. Forensic Sci 1:55–60, 1972

3. Arnason, A, Bjarnason, O: Postmortem changes of human serum esterases. Acta Pathol Microbiol Scand (A) 80:841–846, 1972

4. Bolliger, A, Carrodus, AL: Creatine retention in blood and cerebrospinal fluid. Med J Aust 1:69–72, 1938

5. Brazinsky, JH, Kellenberger, RE: Comparison of immunoglobulin analyses of antemortem and postmortem sera. Am J Clin Pathol 54:622–624, 1970

6. Coe, JI: Postmortem chemistries on human vitreous humor. Am J Clin Pathol 51:741–750, 1969

7. Coe, JI: Use of chemical determinations on vitreous humor in forensic pathology. Int Microfilm J Legal Med, Vol 6, No 3, 1971 Card 9, B–4

8. Coe, JI: Unpublished data on the use of postmortem chemical determinations on blood, cerebrospinal fluid, and vitreous humor presented at the Advanced Forensic Pathology Seminar, American Society of Clinical Pathology, Commission on Continuing Education. Chicago, September, 1971

9. Coe, JI: Use of chemical determinations on vitreous humor in forensic pathology. J Forensic Sci 17:541–546, 1972

10. Co, JI: Postmortem values of thyroxine and thyroid stimulating hormone. J Forensic Sci 18:20–24, 1973

11. Coe, JI: Comparison of antemortem and postmortem serum proteins. Bull Bell Museum Pathobiol 2:40–42, 1973

12. Coe, JI: Further thoughts and observations on postmortem chemistry. Forensic Science Gazette 4:2–6, 1973

13. Coe, JI: Postmortem chemistry: practical considerations and a review of literature. J Forensic Sci 19:13–32, 1974

14. Coe, JI: Postmortem chemistries on blood: particular reference to urea nitrogen, electrolytes and bilirubin. J Forensic Sci 19:33–42, 1974

15. Coe, JI, Sherman, RE: Comparative study of postmortem vitreous humor and blood alcohol. J Forensic Sci 15:185–190, 1970

16. Cooper, WC, Halbert, SP, Manski, WJ: Immunochemical analysis of vitreous and subretinal fluid. Invest Ophthalmol 2:369-377, 1963

17. DeJorge, FB, Jose, NK: Iodine content of normal human eye tissues. Nature 214:491–492, 1967

18. Dito, WR: Transaminase activity in postmortem cerebrospinal fluid. Am J Clin Pathol 42:360–363, 1964

19. Done, AK, Ely, RS, Kelly, VC: Studies of 17-hydroxycorticosteroids: XIV plasma 17-hydroxycorticosteroid concentrations at death in human subjects. Am J Dis Child 96:655–665, 1958

20. Enticknap, JB: Biochemical changes in cadaver sera. J Forensic Med 7:135–146, 1960

21. Enticknap, JB: Lipids in cadaver sera after fatal heart attack. J Clin Pathol 14:496–499, 1961

22. Enticknap, JB: Fatty acid content of cadaver sera in fatal ischemic heart disease. Clin Sci 23:425–431, 1962

23. Erdei, Z, Vass, Z: Chromatographic investigation of free amino acids of the vitreous body. Acta Ophthalmol 45:22–24, 1967

24. Evans, WED: The Chemistry of Death. Charles C Thomas, Springfield, 1963, 100 pp

25. Fekete, JF, Kerenyi, NA: Postmortem blood sugar and blood urea nitrogen determinations. Can Med Assoc J 92:970–973, 1965

26. Felby, S, Olsen, J: Comparative studies of postmortem ethyl alcohol in vitreous humor, blood and muscle. J Forensic Sci 14:93–101, 1969

27. Felby, S, Olsen, J: Comparative studies of postmortem barbiturate and meprobamate in vitreous humor, blood and liver. J Forensic Sci 14:507–514, 1969

28. Finlayson, NB: Blood cortisol in infants and adults: a postmortem study. J Pediatr 67:284–292, 1965

29. Fraschini, F, Muller, E, Zanoboni, A: Postmortem increase of potassium in human cerebrospinal fluid. Nature 98:1208, 1963

30. Gantner, GE, Caffrey, PR, Sturner, WQ: Ascorbic acid levels in the postmortem vitreous humor: their use in the estimation of time of death. J Forensic Med 9:156–159, 1962

31. Glanville, JN: Postmortem serum cholesterol levels. Br Med J 2:1852–1853, 1960

32. Hall, WEB: The medico-legal application of the serum transaminase test. J Forensic Sci 3:117–122, 1958

33. Hamilton, RC: Postmortem blood chemical determinations: a comparison of chemical analyses of blood obtained postmortem with degrees of renal damage. Arch Pathol 26:1135–1143, 1938

34. Hamilton-Paterson, JL, Johnson, EWM: Postmortem glycolysis. J Pathol Bacterial 50:473–482, 1940

35. Hanson, L, Votilla, V, Lindors, R, et al: Potassium content of the vitreous body as an aid in determining the time of death. J Forensic Sci 11:390–394, 1966

36. Hill, E: Significance of dextrose and nondextrose reducing substances in post-mortem blood. Arch Pathol 32:452–473, 1941

37. Hughes, W: Levels of potassium in the vitreous humour after death. Med Sci Law 5:150–156, 1965

38. Jaffe, F.: Chemical postmortem changes in the intra-ocular fluid. J Forensic Sci 7:231–237, 1962

39. Jenkins, WJ: The significance of blood and cerebrospinal fluid urea levels estimated after death. J Clin Pathol 6:110–113, 1953

40. Jensen, O: Postmortem chemical diagnosis of uremia. Proceedings of the Third International Meeting in Forensic Immunology, Medicine, Pathology and Toxicology. London, England, April, 1963

41. Jetter, WW: Postmortem biochemical changes. J Forensic Sci 4:330–341, 1959

42. Jetter, WW, McLean, R: Biochemical changes in body fluids after death. Am J Clin Pathol 13:178–185, 1943

43. Laves, W: Agonal changes in blood serum. J Forensic Med 7:70–73, 1960

44. Leahy, MS, Farber, ER: Postmortem chemistry of human vitreous humor. J Forensic Sci 12:214–222, 1967

45. Leahy, MS, Farber, ER, Meadows, TR: Quantitation of ethyl alcohol in the postmortem vitreous humor. J Forensic Sci 13:498–502, 1968

46. Levonen, E, Raekallio, J, Saikkonen, J: Postmortem determination of blood creatinine and urea. J Forensic Med 10:22–29, 1963

47. Lie, JT: Changes of potassium concentration in the vitreous humor after death. Am J Med Sci 254:136–143, 1967

48. Lindquist, O: Determination of insulin and glucose postmortem. Forensic Sci 2:55–56, 1973

49. Lund, A: Adrenaline and noradrenaline in blood from cases of sudden, natural or violent death. Proceedings of the Third International Meeting in Forensic Immunology, Medicine, Pathology and Toxicology. London, England, April, 1963

50. Mason, JK, Klyne, W, Lennox, B: Potassium levels in the cerebrospinal fluid after death. J Clin Pathol 4:231–233, 1951

51. McCormick, GM: Nonanatomic postmortem techniques: postmortem serology. J Forensic Sci 17:57–62, 1972

52. Mithoefer, JC, Mead, G, Hughes, JMB, et al: A method of distinguishing death due to cardiac arrest from asphyxia. Lancet 2:654–656, 1967

53. Moraru, I, Belis, V, Streja, D, et al: The study of blood cholinesterase in the cadaver in various kinds of death. Proceedings of the Third International Meeting in Forensic Immunology, Medicine, Pathology and Toxicology. London, England, April, 1963

54. Murray, E, Hordynsky, W: Potassium levels in cerebrospinal fluid and their relation to duration of death. J Forensic Sci 3:480–485, 1958

55. Naumann, HN: Urobilinogen in cerebrospinal fluid. Proc Soc Exp Biol Med 65:72–75, 1947

56. Naumann, HN: Diabetes and uremia diagnosed at autopsy by testing cerebrospinal fluid and urine. Arch Pathol 47:70–77, 1949

57. Naumann, HN: Studies on postmortem chemistry. Am J Clin Pathol 20:314–324, 1950

58. Naumann, HN: Postmortem liver function tests. Am J Clin Pathol 26:495–505, 1956

59. Naumann, HN: Cerebrospinal fluid electrolytes after death. Proc Soc Exp Biol Med 98:16–18, 1958

60. Naumann, HN: Postmortem chemistry of the vitreous body in man. Arch Ophthalmol 62:356–363, 1959

61. Naumann, HN: Postmortem diagnosis of insulin shock. JAMA 169:408, 1959

62. Naumann, HN: Personal communication, 1968

63. Naumann, HN, Young, JM: Comparative bilirubin levels in vitreous body, synovial fluid, cerebrospinal fluid and serum after death. Proc Soc Exp Biol Med 105:70–72, 1960

64. Osterberg, K: Personal communication, 1973

65. Patrick, JR: Cardiac or respiratory death, Sudden Infant Death Syndrome. Edited by AB Bergman, JB Beckwith, C Ray. Proceedings of the Second International Conference on Causes of Sudden Death in Infants, University of Washington Press, 1970, p 131

66. Paul, JR: Postmortem blood chemical determinations. Bull Ayer Clin Lab, Penn Hosp 9:51–62, 1925

67. Petty, CS, Lovell, MP, Moore, EJ: Organic phosphorus insecticides and postmortem blood cholinesterase levels. J Forensic Sci 3:226–237, 1958

68. Polayes, SH, Hershey, E, Ledered, M: Postmortem blood chemistry in renal disease. Arch Intern Med 46:283–289, 1930

69. Praetorius, E, Paulsen, H. Dupond, HI: Uric acid, xanthine and hypoxanthine in the cerebrospinal fluid. Scand J Clin Lab Invest 9:133–137, 1957

70. Pucher, G, Burd, L: A preliminary study of the chemistry of postmortem blood and spinal fluid. Bull Buffalo Gen Hosp 3:11–13, 1925

71. Ramu, M, Robinson, AE, Camps, FE: The evaluation of postmortem blood sugar levels and their correlation with the glycogen content of the liver. Med Sci Law 9:23–26, 1969

72. Robinson, DM, Kellenberger, RE: Comparison of electrophoretic analysis of antemortem and postmortem serum. Am J Clin Pathol 38:371–377, 1962

73. Sanders, FW: The preservation of blood for chemical analysis. J Biol Chem 58:1–15, 1923

74. Schlang, HA, Davis, DR: Paper electrophoretic studies of postmortem serum proteins. Am J Med Sci 236:472–474, 1958

75. Schleyer, F: Determinations of the time of death in the early postmortem interval, Methods of Forensic Science, Volume II. Interscience Publishers, John Wiley and Sons, 1963, pp 253-293

76. Scott, W, Root, I, Sanborn, B: The use of vitreous humor for determination of ethyl alcohol in previously embalmed bodies. Presented at the 25th annual meeting of the American Academy of Forensic Sciences, Las Vegas, Nevada, February, 1973

77. Sturner, WQ: The vitreous humor: postmortem potassium changes. Lancet 1:807–808, 1963

78. Sturner, WQ: Postmortem lipid studies: attempts to correlate with death from arteriosclerotic heart disease in the young age group. Forensic Sci Gazette 2:5–7, 1971

79. Sturner. WQ: Postmortem vitreous humor analyses: a review of forensic applications. Forensic Sci Gazette 3:1–4, 1972

80. Sturner, WQ: Magnesium deprivation and sudden unexpected infant death. Letter to the Editor Lancet 2:1150, 1972

81. Sturner, WQ: Personal communication, 1973

82. Sturner, WQ, Coe, JI: Electrolyte imbalance in alcoholic liver disease. J Forensic Sci 18:344–350, 1973

83. Sturner, WQ, Coumbis, RJ: The quantitation of ethyl alcohol in vitreous humor and blood by gas chromatography. Am J Clin Pathol 46:349–351, 1966

84. Sturner, WQ, Dempsey, JL: Sudden infant death: chemical analysis of vitreous humor. J Forensic Sci 18:12–19, 1973

85. Sturner, WQ, Dowdey, ABC, Putnam, RS, et al: Osmolality and other

chemical determinations in postmortem human vitreous humor. J Forensic Sci 17:387–393, 1972

86. Sturner, WQ, Gantner, GE: Postmortem vitreous glucose determination. J Forensic Sci 9:485–491, 1964

87. Sturner, WQ, Gantner, GE: The postmortem interval: a study of potassium in the vitreous humor. Am J Clin Pathol 42:137–144, 1964

88. Sturner, WQ, Putnam, RS: Suicidal insulin poisoning with nine day survival: recovery in bile at autopsy by radioimmunoassay. J Forensic Sci 17:514–521, 1972

89. Tonge, JI, Wannan, JS: The postmortem blood sugar. Med J Aust 1:439–447, 1949

90. Vilstrup, G, Kornerup, J: Protein fractions in corpus vitreum examined by paper electrophoresis. Acta Ophthalmol 33:17–21, 1955

91. Walla, BNS, Sarin GW, Chandra, RI, et al: Preterminal and postmortem changes in serum potassium of children. Lancet 1:1187–1188, 1963

Chapter VI

TIME OF DEATH—TIME OF INJURY

George S. Loquvam, M.D.
Director, Institute of Forensic Sciences
Oakland, California

Introduction

These two points in time can, in certain instances, be vital to the prosecution or defense of a case. Unfortunately, the forensic pathologist does not have, at present, the means to make judgments as precise as he would like in this regard.

The establishment of these two "times" depend primarily on the critical assessment of (1) development of livor mortis, (2) stage of rigor mortis, (3) change of body temperature from loss of heat, (4) amount and state of digestion, and (5) amount of potassium in the ocular fluid. The late changes of putrefaction, age of larvae, presence of molds, state of vegetation beneath the body, and chemical changes in the body fat must also be considered in attempting to estimate the time of death. As Camps has so succinctly put it "it is better to prove, without contradiction, that death could have occurred at a time when a certain person was there, rather than it did occur at some exact moment."

Definitions

Rigor mortis. The stiffening of muscle after death that leads to fixation of joints. Rigor is dependent of the pH of the muscle at the moment of death and the magnitude of the glycogen reserve of the muscle. The pH of the muscle may be altered by antemortem activity and the glycogen reserve determines the pH of the muscle at the onset of rigor.

The onset of rigor, as judged by the fixation of joints, seems to progress from above downwards. When, in fact, what actually is observed, is fixation of joints having less muscle mass controlling them at a rate more rapid than joints having large muscle masses. Examples would be rigor in fingers, toes, and jaw before elbows, and wrist before hip and shoulder.

Livor mortis. This is a mechanical phenomenon occurring after death and results from the effect of gravity on the fluid blood which leads to its settling and collecting in the uncompressed dependent parts of the body. In carbon monoxide poisoning and in some instances of cyanide poisoning, the lividity may be cherry-red in color. If the position of the body is changed after livor has started, the livor may be shifted. If the position of the body is changed after livor is fixed, there may well be fading of the color and shifting to the new dependent position. In an occasional case the change in color and shifting may be used, with caution, to state that the body has been moved after death.*

Body temperature. This is the measured temperature of the body taken by using an accurately calibrated mercury thermometer (or modern electrical recording thermometers with probes may also be employed) and inserting it deep into the rectum, deep into the liver through a stab wound, or using the axillary space.

Ocular fluid. The vitreous fluid removed by means of a small gauge needle and syringe from one or both eyes.

Preliminary Steps

The preliminary steps, of necessity, must be undertaken at the scene before the body has been removed. The environmental temperature, the amount of clothing, the state of nutrition, the evidence of physical activity, if any, and a careful assessment of rigor must all be noted as well as the time these observations were noted. The temperature of the body must also be taken and recorded. The method of taking the temperature is most simply accomplished by inserting the thermometer in the rectal ampulla, letting it equilibrate for at least 5 minutes, and recording the results.

Postmortem Procedures

After the body has been released and taken to the morgue additional observations can be made. Depending on the time interval further assessment must be made of the degree of rigor in relation to the degree found at the scene. The time interval is probably not critical but 4 to 5 hours should elapse to show any significant variation. Be aware that in removing the body from the scene, the attendants may have "broken the rigor;" once a joint has been moved it can no longer be used in assessment of the degree of rigor.

All of the above observations must be included as part of the protocol, as well as the degree and distribution of livor mortis. The secondary observation as to change in temperature and rigor should also be recorded. These observations may be of great value when correlated with other observations supplied to the investigating officers by witnesses.

A careful examination of the food in the stomach and upper small bowel should be made in an attempt to identify particular types of food. There is always the possibility that the time the individual ate this particular food can be documented.

---

* Editors note: Fixation of livor mortis does occur. See Chapter VII for further detail.

Vitreous humor should always be taken at the time of autopsy. Levels of potassium in vitreous humor may be of value if the interval between death and collection is less than 10 hours. It must be stressed that none of these various measurements or determinations is valid by itself in determining the postmortem interval. The more observations made the better chance there is for a reasonable estimate, always remembering it is at best an estimate.

If a considerable length of time has elapsed between death and discovery, other means must be attempted. Collecting fly eggs, larvae, pupae, and adult insects may aid a competent entomologist in estimating the time of formation of these various stages of the insect life cycle. The crushing of plant life beneath the body, the regrowth of plant life and even the growing of small tree shoots through a skeleton can be used to estimate the length of time a decomposing or decomposed skeletonized body has lain in a certain spot.

Time of Injury. One of the frequent questions asked the forensic pathologist by counsel is whether or not the injuries described are contemporary with death. The answer to this type of question is one of the responsibilities of the pathologist and it is incumbent on him to make detailed objective observations in order to express an opinion as to time sequence.

The concept of dating injuries is not new to forensic pathology. However, only one lesion, the subdural hematoma, has been extensively investigated.

The principles involved require careful description of changes in color and the position and extent of lesions. Color photographs may be most useful. In addition, multiple representative microscopic sections must be taken to evaluate the presence and extent of hemorrhage, changes in the erythrocytes, and the presence and extent of inflammatory cells and, in older lesions, the extent of repair as manifested by fibroblastic activity.

As mentioned above, the preliminary steps require accurate descriptions as to color, shape, and size of contusions and abrasions, and examination for evidence of obviously older lesions. The presence or absence of drying and formation of eschar and the color of the surfaces beneath drying crusted areas must be documented.

Before sectioning the area, good color photographs should be taken.

Multiple microscopic sections, carefully documented as to location, are next taken. In the case of subdural hematoma, care must be exercised to insure that the full thickness of the hemorrhage is secured as well as the neomembrane, if present.

Reaction to injury. The phenomenon of aseptic inflammation constitutes the response of the body to injury or death of cells. The degree to which the body responds is proportional to the injury sustained and the time relationship to cessation of vital functions. The need for a clear understanding of sequential events is quite evident. Were the injuries seen on the body contemporary with death? Did they occur after death or hours or days before death?

The initial vascular response is one of capillary dilatation and stasis of blood. The second change to occur is edema of the tissues. The third change is margination of leukocytes in the dilated capillaries and migration of leukocytes into the connective tissue. If the injury is severe enough, there also will be erythrocytes in the tissue. The degree of erythrocytic infiltration is dependent on either the number or size of the blood vessels injured, or both, and the degree of pulse pressure when the vessels were injured.

The amount and degree of infiltration of erythrocytes must be carefully assessed as suffusion of erythrocytes can occur after death especially in areas of postmortem lividity; according to Carscadden[5], margination and emigration of leukocytes may occur up to 30 minutes after death.

In essence then, infiltration of erythrocytes and migration of leukocytes can occur after death. The degree of reaction after death is always less than that occurring before death. It is highly recommended that all forensic pathologists produce sample postmortem wounds, cut microscopic slides and maintain a reference file for comparison in problem cases. Bear in mind, however, that there may, and probably will, be wide variation between cases.

Occasionally, the differentiation between antemortem and postmortem injuries is exceedingly difficult to make. A blow or an injury to a part of a body already altered by postmortem lividity may rupture capillaries distended with blood squeezing some of this blood into tissue spaces mimicking antemortem hemorrhage. In contrast, an antemortem injury sustained when the pulse pressure is near zero, due to other fatal wounds, may show little or no hemorrhage.

Evaluation of emigrated leukocytes must be critically assessed. The number and distribution of leukocytes in a recent hemorrhage will be roughly in proportion to the number in the circulating blood. After an injury polymorphonuclear leukocytes start to appear, first in relation to intact vessels, and then to migrate into areas of hemorrhage. Higgins and Palmer[8] state that these leukocytes begin to disintegrate after 3 to 5 hours and are for the most part completely disintegrated in 21 hours. By 30 hours, the basophilic neutrophile fragments have either undergone autolysis or have been engulfed by phagocytic monocytes.

Migrating monocytes appear between 12 to 24 hours after injury and Maximow[16] states their number is roughly in proportion to the amount of dead tissue present.

Dating the age of subdural hematomas, in our experience, is based on study of 76 cases with well documented traumatic histories and multiple microscopic sections. There are three main points that must be evaluated in a subdural hemorrhage. These are: (1) the status of the erythrocytes

53

in the clot; (2) the development of fibroblasts along the dural side; and (3) the progressive alterations along the arachnoid side.

From 24 to 48 hours the erythrocytes are still easily distinguishable. There may be very early fibroblastic activity at the junction of the clot and the dura, and there is only fibrin on the arachnoid side. At 4 days the erythrocytes start to lose their sharp contour. The fibroblastic layer on the dural side will vary from two to four cells in thickness and there is still only fibrin on the arachnoid side. The difference between a 4-day-old and a 10-day-old subdural hematoma is one of degree. There tends to be laking of erythrocytes and the fibroblasts will vary from 14 to 15 cells in thickness and there probably will be only fibrin on the arachnoid side. In 10 to 15 days, pigment laden histiocytes can be identified. From 15 to 20 days the clot begins to be broken up, by fibroblasts, into islands of poorly preserved erythrocytes and there will be early capillary formation from the dural side. By the twentieth day there are few intact erythrocytes remaining although there may be some fresh hemorrhage from the capillaries present. The dural neomembrane may be one-third to one-half the thickness of the dura and there will be early fibroblastic proliferation along the arachnoid side. By 20 to 25 days, the hematoma will be liquified. The neomembrane will be approximately one-half as thick as the dura and there will be large numbers of pigment laden macrophages throughout the hematoma. By the fortieth day, there will be large dilated capillaries adjacent to the dura. The dural neomembrane will be thick, well organized, and difficult to distinguish from the true dura. The neomembrane on the anachnoid side will likewise be well formed. From 1½ to 3 months there will be hyalinization of the connective tissues present and further accurate dating is probably impossible.

Do's and Don'ts

1. Document by objective description and photography all evidence of trauma.
2. Take adequate microscopic sections of questionable lesions.
3. Take accurate temperature readings of the body and the surroundings in which it is found.
4. Do not attempt to narrowly define time of death on physical evidence only.
5. Do not categorically state an injury is ante- or post mortem without adequate descriptions, photographs and microscopic sections.

References

1. Adelson, L, Sunshine, I, Rushforth, NB: Vitreous potassium concentration as an indicator of the postmortem interval. J Forensic Sci, 8:503–514, 1963
2. Bate-Smith, EC, Bendal, JR: Rigor mortis and adenosinetriphosphate. J Physiol, 106:177–185, 1947
3. Bate-Smith, EC, Bendal, JR: Factors determining the time course of rigor mortis. J Physiol, 110:47–65, 1949

4. Camps, FE: Establishment of the time of death: a critical assessment. J Forensic Sci, 4:73–82, 1959

5. Carscadden, WG: Early inflammatory reactions in tissue following simple surgery. Arch Pathol and Lab Med, 4:329–345, 1927

6. Evans, WE: Adipocere formation in a relatively dry environment. Med Sci Law, 3:145–153, 1963

7. Fiddes, FS, Patton, TD: A percentage method for representing the fall in body temperature after death; theoretical basis of the percentage method. J Forensic Med, 5:2–15, 1958

8. Higgins, GM, Palmer, BM: The origin of fibroblasts within an experimental hematoma. Arch Pathol, 7:63–70, 1929

9. Hughes, WMH: Levels of potassium in the vitreous humour after death Med Sci Law, 5:150–156, 1965

10. Lothe, F: The use of larval infestation in determining time of death. Med Sci Law, 4:113–115, 1964

11. Mant, AK: Adipocere: a review. J Forensic Med, 4:18–35, 1957

12. Marshall, TK: Estimating the time of death: the use of the cooling formula in the study of postmortem body cooling. J Forensic Sci, 7:189–210, 1962

13. Marshall, TK: Estimating the time of death: the use of body temperature in estimating the time of death. J Forensic Sci, 7:211–221, 1962

14. Marshall, TK: Temperature methods of estimating the time of death. Med Sci Law, 5:224–232, 1965

15. Mason, JK, Klyne, W, Lennox, BJ: Potassium levels in the cerebrospinal fluid after death. J Clin Pathol, 4:231–233, 1951

16. Maximow, A: Morphology of the mesenchymal reactions. Arch Pathol Lab Med, 4:557–606, 1927

17. Moritz, AR: Pathology of Trauma. Second edition. Lea and Febiger, Philadelphia, 1954

Chapter VII
POSTMORTEM CHANGES AND ARTIFACTS

Russell S. Fisher, M.D.
Chief Medical Examiner
State of Maryland
Baltimore, Maryland

Introduction

There are regular series of events which occur in the dead body which may shed some light on the time of death or duration of the postmortem interval. These include: the development of lividity, rigidity, postmortem cooling, changes in the chemical constituents of the body fluids, the autolysis of tissue, and the decomposition due to bacterial activity within the body. Further complicating the interpretation of postmortem findings are such events as postmortem trauma, invasion of the body by fly larvae and various other insects, damages to the skin by a variety of invaders, drying of the body, the effects of fire, and finally the artifacts produced by the embalmer in his preparation of the body. Each subject will be dealt with briefly; for more details the reference should be consulted.[1]

Liver mortis. This refers to the purple discoloration of the skin which is caused by accumulation of reduced hemoglobin in the capillaries as it migrates there under the effect of gravity. It will, of course, be absent in those areas where pressure is exerted by the weight of the body on the underlying surface. It may be reddish or cherry pink in carbon monoxide poisoning, cyanide poisoning, and in bodies which are cooled extremely rapidly after death as in thinly clad bodies deposited in snow or very cold water. In the former two, the pinkness is due to chemical changes; in the latter, apparently portions of oxyhemoglobin remain and contribute to the brightness of the color in contrast to the usual dark purple. An associated phenomenon is the so-called "Tardieu's spots"* which are multiple, and frequently confluent, petechiae developing particularly in areas of extensive lividity. They are the result of agonal or postmortem rupture of capillaries with leakage of blood which gradually finds its way to the surface to produce the giant petechiae. Although lividity is variable, it normally begins to form immediately after death and is usually

---

* Editors note: The language purist would apply this term only to subpleural petechial hemorrhages, and not to those located elsewhere.

clearly perceptible within an hour or two. It tends to increase steadily over a period of 4 to 12 hours. In some instances it may become "fixed" due to coagulation of the body fat in the surrounding tissues and therefore remain in a non-dependent position when the body is shifted. Too much importance should not be placed on the "fixation" of lividity since our observations indicate that it may disappear completely from surfaces once they are no longer dependent even though the postmortem interval has been as long as a day or two.

Rigor mortis. This is the hardening of muscle fibers throughout the body resulting from changes in muscle substance with coagulation of the protoplasm. It is the result of increasing acidity and oxygen deficiency and may become manifest within a half-hour after death if the individual has been exercising vigorously or convulsing immediately prior to death. Rigidity builds up over a period of hours, reaching a peak from 4 to 12 hours after death depending largely upon the rapidity of body cooling, the extent of muscular development of the body, and the state of activity prior to death. It may disappear in as little as 9 to 12 hours after death if the body is in an extremely hot environment where decomposition will begin early, and it may persist 3 to 4 days in refrigerated conditions. Once forcibly broken by manipulation the muscle rigidity may stop in its progression in a good many cases, although this is by no means uniform and it may "reset" to some degree. However, once maximal development has been obtained and rigidity is broken it does not recur. Due to the extreme variability very little dependence may be placed upon rigidity as a means of estimating the time of death. It should be borne in mind, however, that the posture of the body at the time it is found, if in the rigid state, must be correlated with the posture into which the body would have collapsed at the time of death. The lack of correlation in such postures suggests that the body was moved after rigidity had its onset.

Body cooling. This is most useful in estimating time of death within the first 4 hours postmortem. There is a general rule that a body cools at 1.5° F per hour when the room temperature is in the neighborhood of 70° and the body is of average fleshiness and is clad in average clothing for such environmental temperatures. The rule, of course, is not applicable under situations where marked temperature variations, wind, or extremes of humidity prevail. The procedure is more useful if serial body temperature at 1 or 2 hourly intervals can be obtained, thus establishing the "cooling curve" which is generally linear in the first several hours. This requires that the environment not be disturbed between the observations.

Postmortem Chemical Changes are discussed in Chapter V (Coe).

Autolysis. Autolysis, of course, can account for a wide gamut of changes, ranging from delicate alterations of individual cells to a complete loss of histologic architecture. Such changes are seen most fre-

57

quently in the pancreas, liver, kidney, gastrointestinal tract, and brain. They are the result of a number of factors including local temperature, rate of development of hypoxia, vascularity, and the presence of autolytic products of metabolism. Early changes are seen so frequently that they soon become readily recognized. The most difficult organ to evaluate grossly is the pancreas. Autolysis with the release of lipolytic and proteolytic enzymes can produce the hemorrhagic, necrotic appearance of acute pancreatitis within two hours after death. Microscopic examination helps differentiate the two conditions based upon the presence or absence of inflammatory reaction.

Association evidence. In addition to the items within the body described above there are frequently evidential items associated with the deceased's habits or environment which help to indicate the time when disability or dying began. Included are: (1) the presence or absence of milk, mail, newspapers or other items usually delivered at identifiable times; (2) whether lights or TV are on or off; (3) the clothing worn by the deceased, night attire, street clothes, etc.; (4) the status of food remnants or dishes and their content which portray meals eaten recently or in preparation; (5) the quantity and location of food in the gastrointestinal tract. Many times the stomach content can be matched with a particular meal eaten at an identifiable time; and (6) in abandoned infant bodies, the clothing, towels, or newspapers in which they are wrapped may serve to identify through laundry marks, as well as to establish the earliest hour at which disposition of the body occurred.

Things that do not happen after death.
1. Exudation of white blood cells.
2. Proliferation of fixed tissue cells.
3. Growth of hair or nails.
4. Penetration of foreign particulate matter to pulmonary alveoli (drowning).
5. Formation of significant carboxyhemoglobin.
6. *Significant degree* of propulsion of food along gastrointestinal tract.

Postmortem trauma. The importance of recognizing the traumatic effects of attempts to resuscitate a dead body cannot be over-estimated in the assessment of death due to blunt injury. Resuscitative efforts may fracture the sternum, ribs, liver, or spleen or may produce pulmonary collapse, subcutaneous emphysema and apparently such unanticipated changes as pulmonary fat, bone marrow, or liver embolism to the lungs when effective cardiac massage has been practiced for some time. Other postmortem injuries such as postmortem stab wounds may also be difficult to distinguish from intra vitam injury. In general postmortem wounds show no hemorrhage or swelling at the margins and by their dry appearance are suggestive that they indeed occur after capillary pressure had reached zero. This may, however, also characterize wounds made during the terminal moments of life in situations of multiple stabbings where the blood pressure falls to low levels before the assailant ceases his repetitive stabbing or cutting of the body. Postmortem blunt injuries, such as occur when an individual may have collapsed and died in the street of natural causes but is subsequently run over by a vehicle, may lead to the accumulation of large amounts of blood in the body cavities and some degree of hemorrhagic infiltration of tissues at the site of gross traumatic lesions. Extreme caution should be exercised in the case of individuals found dead on the highway before concluding that they are victims of hit/run vehicular damage sustained during life rather than postmortem injury after they collapsed from natural causes. The problems become almost impossible to resolve in situations where an individual is hit by a hit/run driver and subsequently run over by other vehicles.

Postmortem invaders. The most common postmortem invader is the blue-bottle fly. There are many varieties of flies, some of which will deposit eggs on living individuals, and indeed, it is not uncommon to encounter maggot infestation in decubitus ulcers and other untreated wounds in marasmic patients. Prior to antisepsis, maggots were used therapeutically to clean up dirty wounds. More commonly, however, maggots deposit their larvae which look like masses of finely grated cheese about the eyelids, about any body orifice and in wounded areas of the body. Some varieties of flies actually deposit live larvae so that they seem to be crawling within a matter of minutes after they are deposited. Most, however, require a period of up to 24 hours to hatch. The larvae then grow rapidly through four or more stages (instars) until they reach maturity at which time they spin a type of cocoon and appear as brown to black oblong bodies, generally not within the body itself but in nearby areas where a warm moist atmosphere will prevail. Eventually, these pupae hatch releasing fully adult flies which are capable of depositing larvae within a few hours after their birth. The duration of the cycle is subject to extreme variation depending on the type of fly but more importantly upon the environment in which the process is occurring. Under optimal conditions the larvae mature from egg to pupa in 6 to 7 days and the pupae hatch in another 6 to 7 days. For further details one should consult an entomologist or Hall's book *Blowflies of North America.*[2] In occasional cases it may be worthwhile to collect larvae from the body and maintain them in a live state until they undergo pupation and hatching as it is easier for the entomologist to identify the species and therefore gross habits if mature larvae and adult forms are available. Additionally, specimens taken at the time of the examination should be fixed in 80 percent alcohol or preferably very rapidly boiling water for minutes and then transferred to 80 percent alcohol for storage. This enables the examiner to estimate the age of the larval growth by study of the specimens. The older larger larvae are most likely to give the true minimal interval between death and the finding of the body; although depending to some extent upon the species, medium or small larvae may in fact be as old as some of the larger specimens found on the same cadaver.

After the fly larvae have come and gone the dermestid beetle invades the body and eats the fibrous and some ligamentous structures. The presence of dermestid beetles in significant numbers usually suggests the body has been dead several months and indeed they may be present for as long as a year or longer if the body has not been completely skeletonized. These beetles are particularly useful in the anatomic preparation laboratory where they clean off undesirable material without destroying bony surfaces or the firm cartilage. (Further information can be obtained from appropriate texts describing this use of the beetle).

Other insects which commonly produce postmortem injuries are roaches and ants. The skin lesions produced by roaches are usually superficial denudation of the epidermis with a rough granulated appearing base and serpiginous outlines. They may, however, be confluent and on occasion when gas gangrene bacterial contamination occurs there may be rapid decomposition due to contamination of the body introduced by the roaches. Antemortem roach bites are recognized and are occasionally the cause of sepsis which originates in skin lesions caused by the biting of the roach. The septic process may include gas gangrene infection. Bodies deposited in sandy locations in warm weather frequently will be invaded by ants which produce multiple superficial areas of injury resembling abrasion and which can be readily confused with abrasions caused by dumping a body on gravelly soil or dragging it across rough terrain. The lack of linear patterning in most ant bites should serve to distinguish them from dragging artifacts.

Both mice and rats will attack the dead body. The lesions induced by mice are readily confused with those produced by roaches but careful examination with a hand lens will usually reveal the fine marks of the rodent incisors. Rat bites and the bites of pet animals feeding on bodies when death occurred in the home and the bite marks of opossum and other animals in the woods may produce extensive postmortem destruction of the body, and indeed, of the bones in areas where the body is extensively destroyed. Such artifacts must not be confused with antemortem trauma.

When death occurs in water a whole series of invaders may produce a variety of artifacts on the body. Leeches which become attached to the skin around the eyes and detach when the body is removed from the water, may produce hemorrhagic lesions simulating a black eye. Similar lesions may develop elsewhere on the body. Crabs and other crustaceans, turtles and fish will all attack the body in the water whether the victim dies of drowning or of other causes and is disposed of in a watery grave. They tend to attack the soft tissues around the eyes, ears, mouth, genitals, and rectum first but, of course, will attack the edges of surface wounds on the body in this same fashion. Injuries from turtles also tend to produce linear wounds that simulate blunt abrasive injuries. In tropical waters, particularly in South America, fish (generally referred to as piranha or caribe) have been known to completely skeletonize a body within a matter of hours due to their flesh-eating habits. Injuries by large fish and sharks have been reported; for further details the reader is referred to Helm's book, *Shark*.[3]

The postmortem injuries associated with fire and which simulate ante-mortem subdural or epidural hemorrhage, antemortem skull fractures and antemortem fractures of the long bones are discussed elsewhere in this manual. (See Chapter XV.)

Postmortem chemical injury. Peculiar artifacts due to drying of the skin after the epidermis has become detached occur in victims who have been exposed to gasoline, coal oil, diesel fuel, and perhaps other solvents. The epithelium detaches on handling the body, and then the underlying dermis turns a peculiar yellow to brown as drying occurs. Such lesions have been confused with antemortem chemical injury or abrasive force. They occur particularly when the body is submerged in water after plane or vehicular crashes but are also encountered in auto-mobile fires when the fire is extinguished with water. Here the combina-tion of wetness and solvent produced provides the necessary exposure to produce the lesions.

Pathologist Induced Artifacts

Postmortem fractures

1. Fracture or preternatural mobility of segments of hyoid bone. In removing the organs of the neck it should be realized that the hyoid, particularly in old people, is often exceedingly fragile and may be easily fractured incident to rough dissection. It should also be borne in mind that osseous union between the segments of the hyoid may be unilateral. Such unilateral mobility or artifact by dissection may lead to the erroneous impression of antemortem fracture. (The writer knows of at least one instance in which a man was found guilty of killing his wife by manual strangulation in which the princi-pal evidence was the report by an inexperienced pathologist that the hyoid bone was fractured).

2. Fractureus of long bones. Elderly or debilitated persons and par-ticularly those who have been confined to bed for a long period of time usually develop osteoporosis with concomitant increase in the fragility of bones. Rough handling of such bones by mortuary assist-ants or hospital orderlies occasionally results in fracture of ribs or of bones of extremities. Such fractures are particularly likely to occur during an attempt to straighten extremities contracted in a state of rigor.

3. Fractures of base of skull. Linear fractures extending into the middle

fossa are frequently produced by the pathologist or by his assistants as an attempt is made to complete the removal of the calvarium by use of a mallet and chisel. Bodies dropped on hard surfaces may also sustain skull fractures.

Intracranial hemorrhage due to artifact. In cases of suspected cranial injury the body should be opened and the cardiovascular system decompressed by opening the heart before the head is opened. If blood has not been drained from the vessels of the head, damage to the dura and the great venous sinuses by the saw may lead to an escape of blood into the subdural space which may simulate an antemortem subdural hematoma. If there is antemortem bruising of the scalp and no other demonstrated cause of death, the erroneous conclusion of death from head injury may result from such an artifact.

Embalming artifacts. The initial stages of embalming with introduction of formaldehyde and other materials incident to pressure injection through the arterial system preserve the tissue well and need not produce significant artifact. However, in most embalmed bodies the second stage consists of "trocharing" the cavities with a long heavy needle connected to suction to dry up excess embalming fluid which may be present in the visceral cavities. This produces all kinds of bizarre puncture wounds and in instances where there may have been antemortem collection of blood it may be disseminated throughout the nearby tissue by the trocharing, making the interpretation of findings extremely difficult.

Do's and Don'ts

1. Visit the scene of death and look for associated evidence in all cases where the length of postmortem interval or time of injury or death may be in question.
2. When pertinent, record the rectal temperature at the onset of the investigation and at intervals thereafter in order to establish the cooling curve and hence the time of death.
3. Look for the tracks of the "silent absent" invaders such as mice, rats, roaches, crabs, fish, turtles, which may explain peculiar lesions on the body surfaces.
4. Collect and properly preserve specimens of larvae, beetles, etc. in appropriate cases.
5. Beware of hasty conclusions of antemortem injury in fire victims where heat artifacts are frequently misleading.
6. Exercise extreme care in removing neck organs to prevent artifactual of the hyoid bone or the thyroid cornua.
7. Do not fail to photograph in both color and black and white all unusual lesions which are not readily and surely identified and refer to consultants who may assist you in correct interpretation of the findings.

62

8. Do not be led into premature guesses of the time of an injury without evaluating all available evidence and taking into account the possible interval of survival from injury to death.
9. Never use mallet and chisel to remove the calvarium if there is a possibility that death may have resulted from cranial injury.
10. Never open the skull in a suspected cranial injury case until the circulation has been decompressed by opening the heart.

References

1. Spitz, WU, Fisher, RS: Medicolegal Investigations of Death. Charles C. Thomas Company, 1973, pp 11–31
2. Hall, DG: The Blowflies of North America. The Thomas Say Foundation and Monumental Printing Company, Baltimore, 1948, 477 pp
3. Helm, T: Shark—Unpredictable Killer of the Sea. Collier Books, New York, New York, 1961, 255 pp

Chapter VIII

IDENTIFICATION

Charles J. Stahl, M.D.
Captain, MC, USN
Armed Forces Institute of Pathology
Washington, D.C.

Introduction

1. The identification of unknown human remains is based upon comparison of known information derived from records with data obtained by examination of the victims.
2. The consultative assistance of other forensic scientists, particularly physical anthropologists, dentists, radiologists, criminalists, and serologists, is often required for conclusive identification.
3. The following records are useful for comparison with the investigative and postmortem findings:
   a. Reports of missing persons
   b. Fingerprints
   c. Dental records
   d. Health records, including past medical history, physical examination, and operative reports
   e. Laboratory records, including blood group and type
   f. Antemortem x-rays
   g. Employment records
   h. Police records
4. The medical examiner or coroner has the responsibility for determining the cause and manner of death, as well as for identifying unknown human remains and estimating the time of death.
5. Accurate identification of unknown human remains is required for the following reasons:
   a. Notification of the next of kin
   b. Completion of official records
   c. Settlement of estates and insurance claims
   d. Use in criminal court proceedings, particularly homicide cases
6. Applications of procedures for identification.
   a. **Antemortem identification**
      (1) Comparative identification of wanted criminals or missing persons

64

(2) Identification of criminal suspects by bite marks

(3) Attempts at interchange of identity

b. **Postmortem identification**

    (1) Identification of single individuals

        (a) Unknown, decomposed, mutilated, skeletonized, or incinerated remains

        (b) Establishment of *corpus delecti* in cases of homicide

    (2) Identification in mass disasters

        (a) Accidental deaths (*i.e.,* fire, explosion, vehicular accidents, aircraft accidents)

        (b) Military operations

    (3) Identification of remains after mass burial or after exhumation of single individuals

7. Objectives of the medicolegal investigation

    a. To determine if the remains are human or non-human

    b. If the remains are human, to estimate the age and living stature, as well as the sex, race, and individual characteristics of the remains

    c. Based upon the investigative and postmortem findings, to provide an estimate of the time of death and/or the duration of time between death and the discovery of the remains

    d. To determine the cause and manner of death

    e. To determine any injuries sustained after death

    f. To determine any indication of interchange of physical evidence between the victim and an assailant

Preliminary Steps

1. **Determination jurisdiction for investigation.**[1]

    a. State or local jurisdiction

        (1) State of local law enforcement agencies

        (2) Medical examiner or coroner

    b. Federal jurisdiction (other than military)

        (1) Federal Aviation Administration (FAA, Federal Aviation Act of 1958)

        (2) National Transportation Safety Board (NTSB)

        (3) Federal Bureau of Investigation (FBI)

    c. Military jurisdiction

        (1) Commanding officer of nearest military installation

        (2) Judge Advocate, or legal officer, of nearest military installation

---

[1] Editors note: Before assuming that jurisdiction is yours, think of the possible ramifications! Especially in mass disasters, many agencies may make conflicting claims as to jurisdiction.

2. **On-the-scene investigation.**

   a. Establish a perimeter around the scene to prevent disturbance of the remains and the physical evidence

   b. Maintain security within the area and require identification procedures for personnel entering the area

   c. Establish and maintain a chain of custody for all physical evidence

   d. Consecutively number the bodies

   e. Provide a system for communicating between investigators on-the-scene and central offices

   f. Maintain the relationship between clothing and personal effects found at the scene and the respective remains

3. **Determine special requirements for facilities and assistance in instances of mass casualties**

   a. Communications

   b. Consecutive numbers and disaster bags for remains

   c. Transportation to remote areas

   d. Facilities for postmortem examination and preservation of remains
      (1) Rental of refrigerated vans
      (2) Building suitable for temporary morgue

   e. Laboratories for examination of physical evidence and/or completion of toxicologic studies, depending upon jurisdiction
      (1) State or local "crime" laboratory
      (2) Medical examiner or coroner
      (3) FBI Laboratory
      (4) Army CID Crime Laboratory
      (5) Military hospital or area laboratory
      (6) Civil Aeromedical Institute (FFA) (commercial carrier or general aviation accidents)
      (7) Armed Forces Institute of Pathology (military aircraft accidents)

   f. Consultants
      (1) Physical anthropologist
      (2) Radiologist
      (3) Dentist
      (4) FIB Disaster Squad
      (5) Identification Division, FBI (Fingerprints)

   g. Support for black and white and/or color photography on-the-scene, as well as during the postmortem examination

   h. Facilities for radiographic studies of remains, including dental x-rays and total body x-rays

   i. Facilities for special studies such as neutron activation analysis

Postmortem Procedures for Identification

1. **Immediate action.**
   a. Obtain all available records for comparison with the results of the examination (Comparison = Identification)
   b. Obtain photographs of remains, clothing, and physical evidence
   c. Obtain selected x-rays, dental x-rays, and/or total body x-rays, as appropriate, for comparison with antemortem x-rays
   d. Obtain fingerprints for comparison with existing records
   e. Obtain samples of hair, blood and body fluids for comparison with known samples of hair and results of prior studies for blood group and type
   f. Obtain consultative assistance, as appropriate, for evaluation and interpretation of skeletal, dental, and radiographic findings
   g. Examine, describe, record, and photograph the clothing and other physical evidence prior to release for other laboratory examinations
   h. Review reports of missing persons, statements of witnesses and next-of-kin in mass disaster situations, and content of passenger manifests provided by representatives of airlines following aircraft accidents

2. **Method for identification**
   a. Least reliable methods
      (1) Personal recognition by relatives or friends
      (2) Clothing [2]
      (3) Personal effects [3]
   b. Scientific methods based upon comparison
      (1) **Fingerprints.** The most reliable method for identification in the United States since the establishment of a national repository for data by the FBI in 1924. Footprints, earprints, and lip prints are also useful provided appropriate records, or records prepared from latent prints, are available for comparison.
      (2) **Dental.** The individual characteristics of teeth, compared with dental records and dental x-rays, provide an excellent means for identification, as well as information concerning the age, race, pre-existing disease, habits, and occupation. Prosthetic appliances are often resistant to the effects of trauma and heat.
      (3) **Skeletal.** Bones are often resistant to the effects of environmental conditions and time, as well as the effects of heat. Depending upon the completeness of the skeletal remains, it is often possible to determine the age at death, sex, race,

---

[2, 3] May be extremely helpful in mass disasters where tentative identification may be partially based upon uniform clothing or unused civilian clothing.

evidence of prior disease or injury, estimate of living stature, and other individual characteristics. Animal bones are distinguishable from human bones.

(4) **Hair.** Microscopic comparative examination of the cuticular patterns and cross sections of hair is helpful in determining race, as well as identifying hair from animals.

(5) **Serologic and cytologic studies.** Blood group determination and Rh typing, animal versus human blood, identification of species, Gm factor, sex chromatin, karyotyping.

(6) **Postmortem examination.** Occupational marks, evidence of preexisting diseases, congenital defects, tattoos, evidence of prior injuries, operative scars and absence of organs due to surgical procedures provide the basis for comparison with medical and employment records.

(7) **Radiographic.** Films obtained during life are compared with postmortem films. Foreign material and metallic fragments, not observed during the postmortem examination, may be detected. Comparison of dental radiographs. Radiographic evaluation of ossification and fusion of epiphyses, as well as of dental development, may provide an estimate of age in children and young adults.

c. Association with or exclusion of remains from other unknown remains based upon individual characteristics, sex, or other factors.

Special Procedures

1. **General**

   a. For each unknown remains, as well as for multiple remains, prepare diagrams and tables for comparison between the unknown and the known features.

   b. Examine eyeglasses, including frames and lenses, for comparison with medical records.

   c. Look beneath eyelids for contact lenses. Examine lenses with ultraviolet light for markings of manufacturer.

   d. If there is a glove-like separation of the epidermis from the hands, the "glove" may be used to obtain fingerprints. If the epidermis is missing, it may be possible to fingerprint the denuded hands. If the hands are putrefied, dessicated, or charred, submit them to the Identification Division of the FBI for further study.

   e. Examine clothing and describe the size, color, condition, and type of each garment. Record descriptions of laundry marks, labels, and name tags. Examine for invisible laundry marks with ultraviolet light.

   f. Remove and examine dentures for name and identification number of individual which may be embedded in the denture base.

68

g. Examine personal effects such as rings, watches, belt buckles, and bracelets for engraved markings. Determine if keys found on the remains provide access to the home or automobile of the missing person.

2. **Teeth.**
   a. Compare antemortem and postmortem dental x-rays and records.
   b. Examine ground sections of teeth microscopically to determine age.

3. **Bones.**
   a. When there is commingling of skeletal remains, examine bones with short wave ultraviolet light to segregate the bones.
   b. Arrange the bones in anatomic order prior to examination.
   c. Obtain photographs and x-rays of osseous lesions for comparison with antemortem films.
   d. Examine pubic bones for parturition pits (indicative of prior pregnancy).
   e. Make an estimate of living stature from accurate measurement of long bones and comparison with tables in textbooks.
   f. Record degree of ossification and fusion of epiphyses for comparison with tables of ossification centers in textbooks.
   g. Examine anterior surface of pubic symphysis in Caucasian male adults for comparison with models for estimate of age.
   h. Microscopically examine ground sections of teeth and cross sections of shafts of long bones for estimate of age.

4. **Hair and Fingernails.**
   a. Obtain samples of known and unknown fingernails and hair for comparison by neutron activation analyses.
   b. Comparative microscopic examination of linear striations of fingernails.

5. **Toxicologic studies.**
   a. Retain tablets or capsules found in stomach for subsequent examination and identification.
   b. Obtain studies, as appropriate, for alcohol, drugs, carbon monoxide, and other toxic agents prior to embalming. Preserve samples by freezing.
   c. In exhumed bodies, obtain samples of soil, water in grave, and fluids in casket for subsequent analysis.

6. **Microscopic examinations.**
   a. Confirm gross pathologic findings.
   b. Distinguish between antemortem and postmortem injuries.
   c. Estimate the age of antemortem injuries by the extent of inflammatory response and reparative processes.

7. **Reconstruction.**
   a. Compare photographs of ears with antemortem photographs.

69

b. Restore the head from the skull and compare with antemortem photographs.

Pitfalls—Do's and Don'ts

1. Establish a perimeter and maintain security during the on-the-scene investigation.
2. Have consecutive numbers for bodies and related personal effects in mass disasters.
3. Establish and maintain a chain of custody for physical evidence.
4. Obtain consultative assistance of physical anthropologists, dentists, radiologists, and other specialists, as indicated.
5. Obtain photographs, x-rays, and other special studies required for identification.
6. Obtain all available records for review and correlation with the investigative and pathologic findings.
7. Examine, describe, record, and tabulate results of examinations for comparison with known information.
8. Do not consider the burned, decomposed, mutilated, or skeletal remains as unsuitable for examination.
9. Do not fail to recognize artifacts and postmortem injuries.
10. Do not attempt to examine commingled skeletal remains. Segregate the bones and arrange in anatomic order.
11. Do not rely upon personal identification by relatives or friends.
12. Do not place specimens for toxicologic studies in formalin solution.
13. Do not confuse the remains of animals with human remains.
14. Do not fail to prepare a contingency plan for a disaster in your community.

References

1. Bass, WM: Recent developments in the identification of human skeletal material. Am J Phys Anthrop 30:459–462, 1969
2. Garn, SM, Rohmann, CG, Silverman, FN: Radiographic standards for postnatal ossification and tooth calcification. Med Radiogr Photogr 43:44–66, 1967
3. Iannarelli, AV: The Iannarelli System of Ear Identification. Police Science Series, The Foundation Press, Inc., Brooklyn, New York, 1964, 168 pp
4. Identication of Deceased Personnel, Department of the Army Technical Manual 10–286. Headquarters, Department of the Army, Washington, DC, January 1964
5. Kerley, ER: Age determination of bone fragments. J Forensic Sci 14:59–67, 1969
6. Krogman, WM: The Human Skeleton in Forensic Medicine. Charles C. Thomas, Springfield, Illinois, 1962, 337 pp
7. McKern, T, Stewart, TD: Skelton Age Changes in Young American Males. Technical Report EP–45, Headquarters, Quartermaster Research and Development Command, Natick, Massachusetts, May 1957, 179 pp
8. Reals, WJ: Medical Investigation of Aviation Accidents. College of American Pathologists, Chicago, 1968, 150 pp

9. Spitz, WU, Sopher, IM, DiMaio, VJM: Medicolegal investigation of a bomb explosion in an automobile: chronological accounts of the explosion in Bel Air, Md, March 9, 1970. J Forensic Sci 15:537–552, 1970

10. Stewart, TD: Evaluation of evidence from the skeleton, Legal Medicine. Edited by RBH Gradwohl. CV Mosby Co, St Louis, 1954, pp 425–427

11. Stewart, TD: Identification by the skeletal structures, Gradwohl's Legal Medicine. Edited by FE Camps. Second Edition. Williams and Wilkins Company, Baltimore, 1968, pp. 123–154

12. Stewart, TD: Personal identification in mass disasters. National Museum of Natural History, Smithsonian Institution, Washington, DC, 1970

13. Suzuki, K, Tsuchihashi, M: Personal identification by means of lip prints. J Forensic Med 17:52–57, 1970

14. Svensson, A, Wendell, O: Techniques of Crime Scene Investigation Second (AM) Edition, Elsevier, New York, 1965, pp 403–411

15. Thomas, F, Baert, H: The longitudinal striation of the human nails as a means of identification. J Forensic Med 14:113–117, 1967

16. Trotter, M, Gleser, GC: Estimation of stature from long bones of American Whites and Negroes. Am J Phys Anthrop 10:463–514, 1952

17. Wecht, CH: The Medico-Legal Autopsy Laws of the Fifty States, The District of Columbia, American Samoa, the Canal Zone, Guam, Puerto Rico, and the Virgin Islands. American Registry of Pathology, Armed Forces Institute of Pathology, Washington, DC, 1971

71

Chapter IX

SUDDEN UNEXPECTED DEATH

John I. Coe, M.D.
Chief Medical Examiner
Hennepin County
Minneapolis, Minnesota

Introduction

Two general types of cases.

1. "Truly" sudden deaths
   a. Occur in seconds to several minutes
   b. Usually observed

2. Unexpected deaths
   a. May be sudden or prolonged
   b. Usually unobserved during terminal period

Autopsy Procedure (See also Chapter I)

1. In either of the above categories, organs should be examined in the following order
   a. Heart, especially the coronary vessels
   b. Lungs and pulmonary arteries
   c. Brain
   d. Larynx and trachea
   e. Remainder of the organs including the aorta, liver, spleen, etc.

2. Rationale for order listed
   a. In over 95 percent of the "truly" sudden deaths and in the majority of unexpected deaths the significant lesion which caused death is found in one of the first three organs listed
   b. When the cause of death is not delineated in 1a, 1b, or 1c above, the pathologist is alerted to the possibility of a difficult case, and then can:
      (1) Examine the remaining organs more carefully
      (2) Save the urine, stomach contents, liver, etc. for toxicologic analysis
      (3) Obtain blood and vitreous humor for postmortem chemistries
      (4) Re-examine the skin for electrical burns, needle marks, etc.

Pathologic Lesions Associated with "Truly" Sudden Death
(In order of most frequent organ involvement)
1. Heart
    a. Ventricular fibrillation
       (1) Coronary sclerosis
       (2) Coronary thrombosis
       (3) Miscellaneous (*e.g.,* aortic stenosis, viral myocarditis, hypertensive myocardiopathy, etc.)
    b. Ruptured acute infarct with tamponade
2. Lungs
    a. Large embolus or thrombus
    b. Air embolism
    c. Massive hemorrhage (*e.g.,* eroded artery)
3. Brain
    a. Massive spontaneous subarachnoid hemorrhage
    b. Primary pontine or cerebellar hemorrhage
4. Larynx
    a. Foreign body obstruction, "Cafe" coronary (not truly natural disease)
    b. Larynogospasm or edema
5. Aorta
    a. Dissecting aneurysm
       (1) Massive acute bleeding from rupture
       (2) Coronary closure from retrograde dissection
    b. Ruptured mycotic or arteriosclerotic aneurysm with massive acute hemorrhage
6. Miscellaneous (*e.g.,* anaphylaxis and other rare and unusual causes)

Pathologic Lesions Associated with Unexpected Death

Many "unexpected" deaths are really cases of medically unattended persons with pathologic abnormalities similar to that observed in routine hospital practice. The lesions found at autopsy indicate that many of these persons must have had symptoms of progressive disease despite the absence of medical attention.[1]

The lesions most frequently found in over 2,000 of the most recently autopsied cases of natural deaths in Hennepin County were as follows
1. Those lesions listed under sudden death (above)
2. Additional frequently found lesions (listed by organ or by organ systems)
    a. Heart, congestive failure from
       (1) Arteriosclerotic heart disease and myocardial infarction
       (2) Rheumatic valvulitis with stenosis and/or insufficiency

---

[1] Editor's note: Some individuals have an extremely high threshold to pain and may not be aware of disease that would cause pain in others.

73

        (3) Bacterial endocarditis
        (4) Alcoholic myocardiopathy
  b. Pulmonary system
        (1) Pneumonia
        (2) Chronic obstructive pulmonary disease
        (3) Tuberculosis
  c. Central nervous system
        (1) Intracerebral hemorrhages or infarcts
        (2) Meningitis
        (3) Brain tumors
        (4) Acute Wernicke's encephalopathy
  d. Gastrointestinal system
        (1) Massive gastrointestinal hemorrhage
           (a) Peptic ulcer
           (b) Esophogeal varices
           (c) Malignancy
        (2) Acute pancreatitis
        (3) Peritonitis
           (a) Perforated ulcer
           (b) Intestinal obstruction—malignancy, incarcerated hernia, post-surgical adhesions, etc.
  e. Genitourinary system
        (1) Acute pyelonephritis with septicemia
        (2) End-stage kidney (glomerulonephritis, chronic pyelonephritis, etc.) with uremia
  f. Miscellaneous
        (1) Carcinomatosis (primary tumors have been found in lung, breast, gastrointestinal tract, pancreas and genital organs)
        (2) Hematopoetic system
           (a) Sickle cell crisis
           (b) Leukemia
        (3) Malignant lymphoma (including Hodgkins disease)
        (4) Septicemia (primary meningiococcemic)

Unexpected Death with Equivocal Anatomic Pathologic Abnormality

1. Severe fatty metamorphosis of liver with or without cirrhosis
  a. Mechanism of death not established
  b. Accepted by forensic pathologists as frequently associated with sudden and unexpected death even in absence of clinical or autopsy evidence of hepatic failure
2. Sudden infant death syndrome (S.I.D.S.) (See Chapter XI)

Sudden or Unexpected Death with No Significant Anatomic Pathologic Abnormalities

1. Biochemical abnormalities
  a. Diabetic acidosis

b. Electrolyte imbalance from vomiting, diarrhea, dehydration, etc.
c. Uremia (prerenal or with equivocal anatomic kidney abnormalities)

Diagnosis in all such cases is made by study of postmortem chemistries of vitreous humor and blood (See Chapter V).

2. Sudden death associated with seizure disorder
   a. Presumptive cause of death based on
      (1) History of epilepsy
      (2) Autopsy evidence of probable seizure
          (a) Loss of sphincter control
          (b) Biting laceration of tongue, cheek, etc.
   b. Probable cause of death based on
      Observation of death during seizure and no other acceptable cause of death demonstrated at autopsy

3. Cardiac arrhythmias of presumptive etiology
   a. Weight reducing medication, presumptive diagnosis made by
      (1) Observation of death as "truly sudden"
      (2) No significant pathologic abnormalities demonstrated at autopsy
      (3) Known use of either
          (a) "Rainbow" type of pill containing thyroid, appetite suppressants, etc.
          (b) Amphetamines or amphetamine-like compounds
   b. Congenital (such as Wolfe-Parkinson-White syndrome) presumptive diagnosis made by
      (1) Observation of death as "truly sudden"
      (2) No significant anatomic pathologic abnormalities
      (3) History of medically established episodes of cardiac arrhythmia

Unexplained Deaths

1. In 5 to 10 percent of all sudden unexpected deaths, there will be no gross anatomic cause of death demonstrated at autopsy. In this situation
   a. Re-examine the heart for evidence of any pathologic abnormality previously overlooked. Take numerous sections from various areas including conducting system for histologic study. Preserve entire heart for further examination
   b. Carefully re-examine the skin for possible lesions overlooked on initial examination (*i.e.,* a small electrical burn, a needle mark in an unexpected location, etc.)
   c. Preserve all of the brain for more complete examination after adequate fixation
   d. Be sure proper material has been collected, properly packaged, and properly labelled for possible toxicologic studies

e. Save blood and the vitreous humor from both eyes for biochemical study (see Chapter V)

f. Review available history (obtain more if possible)

2. After complete gross and microscopic studies, biochemical and toxicologic analyses and review of all available information there will remain a significant percentage of cases in which there is no satisfactory explanation of death. The number of these will depend on

a. Average age of deceased persons in series considered (the younger the average age, the higher the percentage of unexplained deaths)

b. Availability and completeness of support services such as toxicology and biochemistry

c. The willingness of the investigator to accept minimal lesions as deadly

3. In most good medicolegal investigative systems, from 1 to 5 percent of all deaths investigated will remain unexplained

a. In such cases, when investigation indicates that the circumstances are unequivocally those of a natural death, the death certificate can be completed satisfactorily in several possible ways

(1) Cardiac arrhythmia, undetermined etiology

(2) Natural causes

(3) Undetermined, natural circumstances

b. When investigation is equivocal concerning the circumstances, the death certificate should be signed "undetermined" for both the *cause* and *manner* of death (see Chapter III)

Chapter X
INSTANTANEOUS "PHYSIOLOGIC" DEATH

Charles S. Petty, M.D.
Chief Medical Examiner of Dallas County
Director, Southwestern Institute of Forensic Sciences
Dallas, Texas

Such a phrase as "instantaneous 'physiologic' death" is a sharply delimiting one. This is used to describe deaths which are: (1) instantaneous and (2) "physiologic," that is, without a demonstrable morphologic "cause of death."

Actually, no death is "instantaneous" and possibly no person is ever really free of morphologic abnormality. The phrase is used to describe death of a person with no abnormality sufficient to be presumed to have caused the death and where the death is separated by a few seconds (perhaps 5 to 10) from normal life and activity. Every forensic pathologist has encountered instances of death of this type. A typical example from my records follows:

A 17-year-old white girl, apparently in good physical health shop-lifted a small, pocket-sized snapshot album. The theft was noticed and a security guard followed her outside the store, then stopped her and asked that she remove the album from her purse. She handed her babe in arms to her accompanying mother and turned to the guard. The security guard stated "she was looking directly at me and the pupils of her eyes became very large and she dropped to the ground." Mouth-to-mouth artificial respiration administered by the guard was to no avail; resuscitation in the ambulance and at the hospital also failed. No disease process was discovered at autopsy; all organs and viscera appeared normal. Toxicologic examination failed to find any toxic substances in the body tissues and fluids. The mother of the deceased substantiated the statement of the security guard. The brother of the deceased maintained that the guard had "scared her to death." Perhaps he did.

The case presents the essential "negative" findings of instantaneous physiologic death:

1. No trauma
2. No toxin
3. No disease

It also includes the single "positive" feature of instantaneous physiologic death: Witnessed sudden death.

All of the negative and positive findings must be thoroughly examined. The witness must be unimpeachable. (In the instance cited above, all witnesses have an interest in the case, but both "sides" are represented.) The autopsy examination for disease and trauma must be conducted by a person of experience and must be thorough. The toxicologic examination must be conducted by a competent person and also must be thorough. All environmental hazards must be eliminated as possible causes of death.

The case detailed above represents the most "pure" type of instantaneous physiologic death:

No disease, "natural" or "congenital."

No toxin.

No trauma.

Witnessed death.

Age of deceased is that of one not expected to have disease of significance present.

External precipitating cause does not involve actual contact with anything or anyone.

As best can be discerned this death has occurred *de novo*. To be certain, the deceased was under stress. But upon what sort of an organism (psycho-personality) did the stress impinge? Was it an apparently healthy young woman who was frightened with an attendant massive sympathetic nervous system discharge? Or did the stimulus fall upon a carefully guarded (physiologically) young woman whose parasympathetic system was most active? Would ventricular fibrillation be most apt to result in this former milieu, and vasovagal discharge in the latter?

Much has been written regarding the medical, physiologic, psychologic and psychiatric aspects of sudden and unexpected death occurring in individuals with minor or no apparent disease, with and without stress or precipitating cause. The subject matter ranges from highly technical papers in the cardiologic, medical, pathologic, and psychologic literature to highly speculative papers dealing with voodoo deaths and folktales. It is difficult in some of the published papers to distinguish fact from fancy, and because unsubstantiated material is present in many of the writings, there is a tendency for many readers to discount them. Yet more than a thread of truth is present. Highly respectable physicians and scientists have authored many such papers. The true difficulty in regard to instantaneous physiologic death is that there is no morphologic abnormality that can be documented for all to examine. No one can say, at the autopsy table, "this is the arrythmia," or "this is the heart block," or "this represents the vasovagal crisis." After the autopsy, the clinician and pathologist alike wonder why the deceased chose that particular moment to die.

For the forensic pathologist (medical examiner or coroner's pathologist) instantaneous physiologic death is a diagnosis derived more by exclusion than by inclusion. The death certifier must deal with a potpourri of dead individuals and from among them recognize those very few cases of instantaneous physiologic death. He must recognize all cases of overt disease and/or trauma and sift carefully the remaining fraction of deaths so as to assign them their proper cause. Upon this rests many decisions of medicolegal importance (*e.g.,* homicide vs. accident, suicide vs. natural disease process, the proper settlement of estate and insurance questions, and many others). In sifting all types of death situations through the grating of the medicolegal investigation, it would appear that there are several mesh sizes in the sieves proceeding from coarse to fine: the investigation into the circumstances of death, the gross autopsy, the past medical history, the toxicologic examination, x-ray examination, biochemical examination, histologic search, etc. By the time the cases have passed all the various screens, only the possible instantaneous physiologic deaths remain. The more intense and sophisticated the scrutiny, the fewer the cases that can be classified as instantaneous physiologic deaths.

In order to apply the label, instantaneous physiologic death, an intact body with little decomposition must have been available for examination. Without this, the ultimate application of the label "instantaneous physiologic death" is no more than guess work. A second requirement is that the death must have been witnessed. Table I is a general guide to those procedures of elimination which should be applied in every instance.

Before the use of the term instantaneous physiologic death is considered, all of the procedures listed in Table I should have been applied, and no positive findings of significance should have resulted.

*   *   *   *   *   *   *

After the death has been thoroughly investigated, eliminating all apparent causes of death, then some attempt must be made to find "historical" clues which might suggest instantaneous physiologic death. There are two major areas to explore:

1. Vasovagal reflex (inhibition)
   In this situation, a history of a precipitating event will be developed and possibly a history of vasovagal episodes of lesser degree may be elicited from relatives and friends of the deceased. Since the flood of reflex activity of this nature is initiated by an "external cause," the precipitating event (if the death was witnessed) will likely be recalled (*e.g.,* a minor blow to the neck, epigastrium, precordium, puncture of the pleura, or penetration of the cervical os or urethra by instrument; pressure on the carotid sinus; etc.). Collapse occurs immediately, and death is quick to occur. Probably the heart slows, then stops, and death results from asystole.

79

TABLE I.

	To Eliminate
Natural disease	History —medical
	Autopsy—gross
	—microscopic
	Bacteriologic examination
Trauma	History —circumstance of death
	Autopsy—gross
	—microscopic
	X-ray examination
Toxins and poisons	History —circumstance of death
	—occupation
	—drugs and toxins available
	Autopsy—gross
	—microscopic
	Toxicologic examination
	Biochemical examination
Biochemical disturbances	Biochemical examination
	Vitreous humor examination
	Blood examination
	Urine examination

Elimination pocedures applicable to death investigation. (Others may be considered and added.) If all of these suggested approaches fail to develop leads to the actual death cause, instantaneous physiologic death may be considered as a proper term to be used to certify the cause of death.

2. Ventricular fibrilation
   No precipitating event is necessary although there may be one. History of fainting may be elicited from family and friends of the deceased. Such may have occurred when the individual was very tired and under great emotional strain. Death is from "spontaneous" ventricular fibrillation.

3. A combination of the two, vasovagal reflex and ventricular fibrillation, may be possible in theory and may actually take place (*e.g.,* cases of myocardial damage resulting from disease with an overlay of external or precipitating causes). But in such an instance, a disease process would be noted at the time of autopsy, and the diagnosis of instantaneous physiologic death would be unnecessary.

* * * * * *

How does the medicolegal officer certify the death? The type of the instantaneous physiologic death may be well enough defined so as to state on the death certificate:

1. Fatal ventricular fibrillation (when there is a history of preceding syncope due to arrhythmia).

2. Vasovagal reflex upon thoracentesis.

Both of the choices demand that the body be available for autopsy without undo delay, and that the death be witnessed. Many deaths, however, are not witnessed, and despite a negative autopsy, etc., all that can be said on the death certificate is: "Cause of death not ascertained upon autopsy and toxicologic examination."

In point of practicality it should be noted that frequently minor disease enters the picture and Table II gives the possibilities which may be considered.

If you desire some fascinating reading the following bibliography is offered as an introduction.

TABLE II.

Disease	Cause	Certification
1. None	None	tendency to certify:
2. None	Precipitating present*	"cause of death—undetermined"
3. Minor cardiac	Precipitating present*	tendency to certify:
4. Minor cardiac	None	"death due to disease—natural causes"

* May be pressure to put precipitating cause on the death certificate and certify as an accident

An overview of different methods (philosophies) of certifying the cause of death in instances where disease is absent or present in minimal (apparently sublethal) amounts.

References

1. Adelson, L: anatomic cause of death. Conn State Med J 18:732–(739, 1954

2. Goldstein, S: Sudden Death and Coronary Heart Disease. Futura, Mt. Kisco, 1974, 213 pp

3. Kayssi, AI: Death from inhibition, and its relation to shock. Brit Med J 2:131–134, 1948

4. Moritz, AR, Zambeck, N: Sudden and unexpected deaths of young soldiers. Arch Pathol 42:459–494, 1946

5. Pruitt, RD: On sudden death. Am Heart J 68:111–118, 1964

6. Pruitt, RD: Death as an expression of functional disease. Mayo Clin Proc 49:627–634, 1974

7. Richter, CP: On the phenomenon of sudden death in animals and man. Psychosomatic Med 19:191–198, 1957

8. Simpson, K: Modern Trends in Forensic Medicine. CV Mosby Co, St Louis, 1953 pp 59–79

9. Wallace, WA, Yu, PN: Sudden death and the pre-hospital phase of acute myocardial infarction. Ann Review Med 26:1–7, 1975

10. Weiss, S: Instantaneous "physiologic" death. New Engl J Med 223:793–797, 1949

11. Wright, KEJr, McIntosh, HD: Syncope: a review of pathophysiological mechanisms. Prog Cardiovasc Dis 13:580–594, 1971

"Psychologic" Stress References

1. Brod, J, Fencl, V, Hejl, Z, et al: Circulatory changes underlying blood pressure elevation during acute emotional stress (mental arithmetic) in normotensive and hypertensive subjects. Clin Sci 18:269–279, 1959

2. Engel, GL: Sudden and rapid death during psychological stress. Folklore or folk wisdom? Ann Intern Med 74:771–782, 1971

3. Gazes, PC, Sovell, BF, Dellastatious, JW: Continuous radioelectrocardiographic monitoring of football and basketball coaches during games. Am Heart J 78:509–512, 1969

4. Hanson, JS, Tabakin, BS: Electrocardiographic telemetry in skiers. Anticipatory and recovery heart rate during competition. New Engl J Med 271:181–185, 1964

5. Malik, MAO: Emotional stress as a precipitating factor in sudden death due to coronary insufficiency. J Forensic Sci 18:47–52, 1973

6. Moss, AJ, Wynar, B: Tachycardia in house officers presenting cases at grand rounds. Ann Intern Med 72:255–256, 1970

7. Sharpey-Schafer, EP, Hayter, CJ, Barlow, ED: Mechanism of acute hypotension from fear or nausea. Brit Med J 8:878–880, 1958

8. Simonson, E, Baker, C, Burns, N, et al: Cardiovascular stress (electrocardiographic changes) produced by driving an automobile. Am Heart J 75:125–135, 1968

82

Chapter XI

SUDDEN INFANT DEATH SYNDROME: CRIB DEATHS

Jerry T. Francisco, M.D.
Chief Medical Examiner
State of Tennessee
Memphis, Tennessee
and
Charles S. Hirsch, M.D.
Associate Pathologist and Deputy Coroner
Cuyahoga County Coroner's Office
Cleveland, Ohio

Introduction

1. **Definition.** The sudden unexpected death of an apparently healthy infant usually between 6 weeks and 6 months of age, in which a complete autopsy fails to reveal an obvious or recognizable cause of death and a careful investigation of the circumstances surrounding the death fails to provide suspicion of an unnatural manner of death.

2. **Epidemiology.** This syndrome claims approximately three babies of every 1,000 live births, with a slight preponderance of males and a higher frequency occurring in lower socioeconomic groups. The peak incidence is in ages 2 to 4 months and 75 percent of the deaths are of infants less than 6 months old. Such deaths rarely happen in infants less than 2 weeks or more than 9 months old. Occurrence after 1 year of age is doubtful.

   These deaths occur throughout the year but usually are more frequently recorded during the cold months.

3. **History.** The majority of victims are found, in a prone position, in their cribs in the morning. Apparently they die rapidly during sleep and do not cry or have audible respiratory distress. Almost half of them have had a minor upper respiratory infection ("cold" or "sniffles") in the week or two preceding death. Typically, they are robust, well-fed, clean infants who appear to be entirely normal prior to their unanticipated deaths.

4. **Cause.** The cause of this syndrome is not known, and there is no generally accepted theory. It is rare to have more than one occurrence in a family. However, episodes where both twins were found

83

dead at the same time have been recorded and tend to implicate some developmental problems common to both.

If the autopsy of an infant reveals a cause of death (*e.g.,* suppurative meningitis, or previously unrecognized pathologically significant congenital anomaly), the case in question is not an example of the "sudden infant death syndrome."

Preliminary Steps

1. Familiarize yourself with the available information concerning the baby's history and the circumstances surrounding the death. Is there any suspicion that the child may have hanged himself, compressed his neck between the slats of a defective crib, suffocated from a plastic bag clinging to the face and covering the airway, or been the victim of traumatic asphyxia resulting from overlying?
2. If the infant is unusually dirty, bruised, or malnourished, consider the possibility of fatal child abuse.[1] In this instance, take photographs and x-rays of the entire baby prior to beginning the autopsy. Have the blood tested for salicylates and commonly available sedative drugs if there is anything suspicious about the circumstances, appearance of the child or autopsy findings.
3. The possibility of carbon monoxide intoxication should be considered. Infants will accumulate carbon monoxide more rapidly than adults when breathing the same contaminated air. Thus, they will reach a fatal level of carboxyhemoglobin more rapidly than adults. The adult may have few symptoms while the infant may already be dead.
4. A visit to the scene of death by a competent observer prior to commencing the autopsy may be of great help.

Autopsy

1. The autopsy should be complete, including examination of the brain and neck organs. Its purpose is to exclude injury or demonstrable disease as the cause of death.
2. Characteristic gross anatomic findings in the sudden infant death syndrome include:
   a. pulmonary congestion and edema sometimes with froth in the airways
   b. petechiae of the epicardium, pleurae, and thoracic thymus
   c. *terminal* aspiration of gastric content
3. Microscopically, there is a variable lymphocytic infiltrate in the submucosa of the respiratory passages and pulmonary interstitium, which is indistinguishable from the histologic appearance of the same tissues taken from control infants (*e.g.,* those suddenly killed in automobile crashes). Step sections of the larynx perpendicularly oriented to the

---

[1] Editor's note: Remember that in some instances, the baby may have been "battered" without visible external injury.

plane of the laryngeal ventricle, frequently show peculiar, focal degeneration and inflammation within the stroma or mucosa, or both, of the true vocal cord. The significance of the latter observation is unknown and the presence of such does not prove "sudden infant death syndrome."

Pitfalls and Pearls

1. These infants do not suffocate in bedding, and they do not die by aspirating gastric content. Terminal or agonal regurgitation and aspiration of gastric contents occurs frequently; it occurs because the infant is dying and is not the cause of death. Fatal overlying, compression of the infant's trunk by a sleeping adult or sibling is possible, but this diagnosis is untenable unless there is a compelling history and physical evidence (not simply the presence of another person sleeping in the same bed). Status thymicolymphaticus was a fatal mechanism conjured out of a misinterpretation of normal anatomy, and fatal "whiplash" injury of the cervical vertebral column does not cause the sudden infant death syndrome. In summary, there is no reasonable mechanical explanation for these deaths.

2. Postmortem refrigeration of infants frequently congeals the subcutaneous fat in a fashion that leaves a conspicuous crease where there was a normal skin fold of the neck. This can be misinterpreted as the mark of a ligature (strangulation) if one fails to notice that the furrow is an exaggeration of a natural crease and is neither abraded or contused.

3. Nasal and perioral abrasions, caused by resuscitation attempts, can be misinterpreted as signs of smothering. Also, visceral laceration and head injuries are occasionally inflicted during vigorous resuscitation. Prior to concluding that an infant has been smothered or has died as a result of some other recent injury, be certain to exclude trauma caused by resuscitation. This requires specific inquiry (parents, hospital personnel, ambulance attendants, firemen, police officers) and is not accomplished by a naive reliance upon the notation "DOA" to assume that nobody attempted to revive the infant.

4. Do not neglect the psychologic (parental) and social aspects of the problem. Many parents blame themselves for the infant's death, and many are left with a legacy of guilt. It is desirable that the parents receive prompt verbal and written communication stressing that:
   a. The infant died of "natural causes"
   b. The infant's death was neither predictable nor preventable
   c. The infant did not die because the parents did something wrong or because the parents failed to do something that they should have done.
   d. Future offspring will not necessarily die as did this one

5. Referral of the parents to a local or state chapter of the National

85

288-953 O - 79 - 7

Foundation for Sudden Infant Death or International Guild for Infant Survival helps to provide additional information and support for the grieving parents. (To learn more about these organizations, you may write: National Foundation for Sudden Infant Death, Inc., 1501 Broadway, New York, New York 10036 or International Guild for Infant Survival, 7501 Liberty Road, Baltimore, Maryland 21207.

References

What is not known about "sudden infant death syndrome" seems to outweigh what is known. With the increasing interest of others than those involved in forensic medicine, there have been many recent publications.

Still one of the very best, although much out of date, is: Wedgewood, RJ, Benditt, EP: *Sudden Death in Infants: Proceedings of a Conference on Cause of Sudden Death in Infants, September 1963, Seattle, Washington.* Public Health Service Publication 1412, Government Printing Office, Washington, DC, 1966, 165 pp

An update of this, the report of the 1969 conference, also held in Seattle, is: Bergman, AB, Beckwith, JB, Ray, CG: *Sudden Infant Death Syndrome.* University of Washington Press, Seattle, 1970, 248 pp

A more recent conference, this time held in England, is dated 1970: Camps, FE, Carpenter, RG: *Sudden and Unexpected Deaths in Infancy (Cot Deaths).* Wright, Bristol, 192, 129 pp

Two other references may be particularly useful: Valdes-Dapena, M: "Sudden and unexpected death in infancy: a review of the world literature 1954-1966." Pediatrics 39:123-138, 1967 Sturner, WQ: "Sudden unexpected infant death," Legal Medicine Annual-1971. Edited by CH Wecht. Appleton-Century-Crofts, New York, 1971, pp 47-66.

There has been no breakthrough in the understanding of the waste basket into which the forensic pathologist places all cases of infant deaths he investigates, having eliminated all instances of death due to provable, known trauma or disease. The more carefully each case of infant death is worked up from the investigational, pathologic, toxicologic, immunologic, and all other phases, the lower the percentage of sudden infant death syndrome in any given series.

Chapter XII
THE BATTERED CHILD

George S. Loquvam, M.D.
Director, Institute of Forensic Sciences
Oakland, California

Introduction

The autopsy of "the battered child" like the autopsy of any victim of a known or suspected homicide, must, in addition to being surgically complete, be supported for the present record and future reference (court) by photographs, x-rays, and microscopic sections of all pertinent lesions. These records preserve in graphic form not only the lesions themselves but assist in the establishment of the sometimes all important time and environmental factors.

The original observations of Caffey[2] regarding the association of subdural hematomas and of fractures of longbones in children stimulated a number of articles concerned with this apparently rare and, at that time, unexplainable syndrome. It was not until the early 1960's that Kempe[4] coined the term "the battered child syndrome" and presented two condensed case histories depicting some of the problems encountered in dealing with this syndrome. There appeared in the late 1960's a book, edited by Helfer and Kempe,[3] dealing in detail with the history, incidence, and medical, psychiatric, social and legal aspects of this syndrome.* Inasmuch as this presentation deals only with the forensic pathology aspects of this problem, the reader is referred to this excellent monograph for the other areas covered.

Definition. For the purposes of this chapter the "battered child" is considered to be the victim of repeated assaults with death resulting. Excluded here are single trauma homicides, child neglect, etc.

Incidence. The Coroner's Office of Alameda County, California (population 1,500,000) investigated during the 12-year span (1960 through 1971) 51 fatal cases of child batterings. See Tables I and II for details.

In 1965, a registry of child abuse was established in California.[1] During the first 5 months of operation, approximately 489 incidents

---

* Editors note: This book is now in a second edition (1974). Same title, same publisher.

TABLE I. *Incidence of Battered Children by Age, Sex and Race—Alameda County, California 1960–1971*

Age	Number
0–6 months	15
6–12 months	15
12–18 months	6
18–24 months	2
2–5 years	9
5–10 years	2
Unstated	2
	51
Sex	
Male	29
Female	22
	51
Race	
White	24
Black	26
Other	1
	51

TABLE II. *Battered Children with History at Variance with Findings in 37 Cases*

Findings	Number
Old injury	14
Old fracture	15
Site of Injury	
Head	27
Abdomen	13
Structures Injured	
Single organ	10
Multiple organs	3
Fractured neck	3
Fractured pelvis	1
Other Causes of Death	
Drowning	1
Aspiration with blunt injury	1
Suffocation	1
Stabbing	1
Fat emboli	2

of physical abuse of children were reported from the entire state. From this, it can be estimated that there would be approximately 1200 instances of physical abuse of children during a single year in California. Of this total number, approximately 5 percent fit the "battered child syndrome" although fewer than 1.5 percent of the victims died.

Preliminary Examinations

As in all facets of forensic pathology, the pathologist, of necessity, must have an inquiring mind and a high index of suspicion. The need for suspicion or skepticism is amply substantiated by the fact that in three-fourths of the Alameda County cases there was complete disparity between the history and the findings at autopsy.

Typical histories recount: falls from highchairs; stumbling and falling downstairs; fall from bed; burns resulting from child's having pulled pan of boiling water off stove, etc.

As has been frequently stated, "the autopsy is the last step in a medicolegal investigation." Before a pathologist can logically approach the problem of "the battered child," he must carefully investigate all of the circumstances surrounding the death. In many jurisdictions, this is capably handled by trained investigators. In other areas of the country, this investigation may be inadequately performed or not performed at all. In these areas, the pathologist must conduct his own investigation and, by example, train the responsible investigative agents to collect and report the essential pertinent data.

Regardless of how the investigation is conducted, it is incumbent for the pathologist to secure all the information possible before starting his examination. As stated above, the histories in three-fourths of our cases were completely misleading as to the circumstances surrounding the death. In general, all childhood deaths are suspected of fitting into this category until trauma is eliminated at the time of autopsy as a cause of death. This necessitates an investigation by the medical examiner or coroner and by the appropriate police department and social service agency.

Postmortem Examination

The postmortem examination should begin with a general description of the body documenting the age, length, weight, state of nutrition, identifying marks, color of hair, color of eyes, and general cleanliness of the body and clothing. In the instance of an infant in diapers, this would include care as manifested by degree of diaper rash, secondary infection in diaper area, scarring and skin change. The presence of insect infestation, burn scars, swelling of joints, asymmetry of head or extremities, and congenital defects should be described. All evidence of external injury must be anatomically located, measured, and carefully recorded. To document the injuries described, suitable color photographs must be taken with identifying label and some measuring device. The photographs must be taken close enough to show the lesions and a readily identifiable anatomic landmark so that they can be orientated at a later date. In some instances, black and white photographs using orthochromatic film must be taken to show bruising that may not be as evident in color photographs.

The bodies may be screened by fluoroscopic examination where available if the examiner is competent in the technic. However, if evidence of old or recent injuries is found, this must be documented by x-ray, preferably a complete body survey, for future courtroom presentation.

A complete autopsy including head, neck, chest and abdomen must be performed.

Head. The usual inter-mastoidal incision may well be employed with careful description of any hemorrhage found in scalp or galea aponeurotica. Color photographs should be taken to document the presence and extent of hemorrhage, both old and recent. Microscopic sections should be taken for age-dating of lesions. Skull fractures must be described (both before and after removal of calvarium) documenting locations, shapes, and extent. Careful description of epidural, subdural, and subarachnoid hemorrhage must be made to include amount, position in relation to fractures, color and adhesiveness, or lack of it. Careful microscopic study of subdural hemorrhages, including adjacent normal or uninvolved dura, are often useful for age-dating. Frequently a history of a fall or repeated falls is given. The careful differentiation between coup and contrecoup lesions of the brain will, of course, assist in determining whether the injury resulted from a moving head striking a fixed object or a moving object striking a fixed head.

Neck. The neck organs should be removed from the floor of the mouth distally and a careful search made for foreign body or inflammatory obstruction of the airway. Trauma of any sort to the hyoid bone, the cartilages of the larynx, or the soft tissues must be well documented.

Chest and abdomen. As in any autopsy, the organs must be described and weighed, and note made of the presence (including volume) or absence of fluid in any of the body cavities. It is very important to note any old or recent fractures of the vertebral bodies or ribs. Sections must be made of all sites of fracture and of all organs. Lacerations of the pancreas, tearing into the round ligament at its insertion into the liver, mesenteric hemorrhages, and contusions of small and large bowel are frequent findings in cases of blunt injury to the abdomen.

Extremities. Asymmetry of arms or legs should be examined by x-ray first and then by incision, removal of injured bone segments is frequently necessary. Incision into asymmetrical buttocks may show massive tissue destruction and hemorrhage due to blunt trauma. Examination by frozen section for fat embolism may be of value whenever there is large destruction of tissue such as in and around the buttocks or in bone fractures. The soles of the feet should be examined for possible occult trauma.

Toxicology. Adequate specimens for toxicologic examination must be taken. These include: (a) 10 to 15 ml. clotted blood; (b) all urine; (c) one kidney; (d) 50 gms. liver; and (e) stomach contents. These specimens must be taken in chemically clean containers, adequately labelled, and the chain of possession carefully maintained. In selected cases, it may be necessary to take hair samples with root structures, fingernail clippings, and 50 gms. of brain.

Bacteriology. If infectious disease is suspected, specimens for heart blood culture, lung culture, and spinal fluid cultures may be necessary to establish the etiologic agent causing or contributing to death.

Editor's comment. When all factual information concerning the circumstances is available and the autopsy is complete, an opinion as to cause and manner of death should be prepared in order that the law enforcement agencies may take appropriate action.

References

1. Bureau of Criminal Investigation and Identification, State Department of Justice, Sacramento, California

2. Caffey, J: Multiple fractures in the long bones of infants suffering from chronic subdural hematoma. Am J Roentgenol, 56:163–173, 1946

3. Helfer, RE, Kempe, CH: The Battered Child. University of Chicago Press, Chicago, 1968, 268 pp

4. Kempe, CH, Silverman, FN, Steele, BF: The battered-child syndrome. JAMA 181:17–24, 1962

Chapter XIII
RAPE

The Forensic Pathology Committee
College of American Pathologists

Introduction

1. Forcible rape may be defined as unlawful sexual activity with a female against her will (without consent) using force or deception.
2. Victims of rape may be any age. Severe genital injury is characteristically seen when the victim is a child or an elderly woman; such injury is not common in mature premenopausal women (who may be accustomed to sexual intercourse).
3. Victims of fatal altercations between homosexuals should be examined using the same technics as those used to examine female victims of rape.
4. Victims of rape-murder and homosexual murder frequently show evidence of extreme violence (overkill).[1] Females are often killed by strangulation; multiple causes of death are not unusual.
5. Objectives of the medicolegal autopsy in instances of rape-murder are:
   a. To determine the cause of death
   b. To confirm sexual activity by demonstration of sperm, acid phosphatase
   c. To determine associated chemical factors (*i.e.,* alcohol, drugs)
   d. To determine any physical violence (*e.g.,* genital, general)
   e. To obtain specimens for examination in the laboratory (*e.g.,* fingernail clippings or scrapings, clothing, pubic hair, head hair, and vaginal, rectal, and oral swabs and washings)

Preliminary Steps

1. The victim should be photographed with clothing as it was at the time of discovery. This will document the position and condition of the garments (*e.g.,* skirt pulled up to the level of mid-abdomen and torn panties around one ankle). Description of the clothing and the condition of the body when first viewed by the prosector should comprise the first segment of the autopsy protocol.

---

[1] Editors Note: This implies trauma by several mechanisms, and/or excessive and repetitious use of the murder weapon or weapons.

2. Undress the body on an undercovering such as a freshly laundered sheet, disposable plastic or paper sheet, or fresh roll paper. All foreign objects remaining on the undercovering after the body is undressed should be retained and examined for trace evidence (see Chapter IV). Do not cut or tear clothing when undressing the ·body.
3. Comb the pubic hair for loose or foreign hair.
4. Obtain samples of pubic and scalp hair with roots. (This is accomplished by plucking rather than shaving or cutting the hair.)
5. Clip off the free ends of the fingernails or scrape the under-surface of the free ends with a dull object and retain nail clippings or scrapings for examination. When the fingernails are broken, document this finding by photograph as this is an important observation.
6. Use a vaginal speculum and good light to examine the vagina and uterine cervix.
7. Obtain vaginal swabs and aspirates; make smears on labelled microscopic slides.
   a. Examine an unstained hanging drop preparation for motile sperm.
   b. Fix the smears at once so as to prevent further damage and alteration of sperm by slow drying.
   c. Prepare stained slides (hematoxylin and eosin, Papanicolaou's or any other which you may prefer) and retain permanently. Gram stain may be useful to show gonococcal organisms.
   d. A culture for gonococcal organisms should be made. This may be a useful adjunct.
   e. Vaginal aspirates should be examined for acid phosphatase activity. If the vagina appears dry, use a small amount of saline for irrigation. If an excess of material is present on the vaginal swabs used for making microscopic slides, place the swabs in a clean test tube and seal. These swabs are a good specimen to test for acid phosphatase activity.[2]
8. Swab the mouth (including pharynx) and rectum and examine the swabs for the presence of sperm and acid phosphatase (as with vaginal specimens).
9. Suspicious stains from the vulva, thighs, or other areas should be collected by swabbing to examine for the presence of sperm and acid phosphatase. If such stains are dry, scrape them from the

_____

[2] Editors note: Such swabs may also be useful to examine for blood group substances (A,B,O). The seminal fluid may be typed in approximately 80 percent of the cases as approximately 80 percent of individuals will secrete their blood group substance into their body fluids including seminal fluid.

If seminal fluid typing is a goal of the examination of the possible rape-victim, a specimen of saliva or other body fluid should be obtained so as to determine the secretor-status of the deceased. This will avoid mistaking her (his) blood group substance for the rapist's (or other sex-crime type).

surface with a clean scalpel blade. Seminal stains fluoresce with ultraviolet light, but not all stains which fluoresce are semen.

10. Photographs
    a. Identification of victim ("mug shot").
    b. Injuries—if obscured by dried blood, these photographs have limited or no value.
    c. Identification or autopsy number and scale of size should be included in each photograph.

Autopsy

1. Do not fail to do a complete autopsy including the head and neck.
2. Specimens to be saved:
    a. Blood for typing and toxicologic analyses.
    b. Plucked hair samples from head and pubis.
    c. Fingernail clippings or scrapings.
    d. Vaginal, anal (rectal), oral, or other swabs as indicated.
    e. Urine, bile, gastric content or other appropriate specimens for toxicologic analyses.
3. Note the composition of stomach contents; this may help to determine the time of death (see Chapter VI).
4. Document all injuries and associated natural disease.

Special Procedures

1. Each article of clothing should be inventoried, air dried if wet, and placed in an individual bag or container.
2. Do not tear or cut the clothing.
3. Seminal stains fluoresce in ultraviolet light, but fluorescence of stains is not pathognomonic of semen. Chemical demonstration of acid phosphatase or identification of sperm is required to confirm the identification of seminal stains.
4. Bloodstains on clothing should be typed to determine whether they are from the victim or possible assailant.
5. Foreign hair or other trace evidence from clothing or the body should be carefully examined and retained.

Pitfalls and Pearls

1. Keep strict criteria for the identification of sperm.
    a. Head, neck and tail must be present to identify a sperm; fragments are not diagnostic.
    b. At least two sperm must be identified.
    c. Beware of confusing trichomonads, fibers, leukocytes, and degenerating epithelial cells with actual sperm.
2. Evidence of recent sexual intercourse is not proof of rape when the victim is a mature woman.
3. Consider any female dead of violence as a potential victim of rape;

a strangled woman should be considered a victim of rape until proven otherwise.

4. Think of homosexuality when there is obvious excessive trauma to a male victim of homicide.

5. Severe injury of the vagina or uterine cervix in a mature woman is not characteristic of rape. Such findings suggest that a foreign object (*e.g.,* broomstick, bottle, etc.) has been introduced forcibly into the vagina.

6. Acid phophatase activity should be strongly positive to indicate the presence of semen. If it is strongly positive but sperm are not identified on smears, re-examine these smears.

   a. If the post-intercourse interval (antemortem, postmortem, or both) is sufficiently long, there may be no remaining intact sperm in the vagina.

   b. The sexual partner (or assailant) may have had no sperm in his ejaculate (*e.g.,* primary disease of the testes or ducts; successful vasectomy, in which case sperm will be absent from the ejaculate within 6 to 8 weeks post operative; post suprapubic prostatectomy; or a sexually immature male).

7. Approximately 80 percent of men are secretors of blood group substances in their semen. Seminal stains on clothing or vaginal aspirates may be suitable to determine the blood group of the assailant.

Editor's Comment: Ordinarily the pathologist (or medical examiner) will not be concerned with the examination of the living alleged victim of criminal sexual assault; however, not infrequently the coroner or coroner's physician is responsible for the proper examination of alleged victims of rape. Because of the usefulness of the American College of Obstetricians and Gynecologists Technical Bulletin Number 14, which deals with suspected rape, this Bulletin is reproduced in its entirety on the following pages (with the kind permission of the College). It is hoped that the ready availability of this article will prove useful to pathologists and physicians generally).

References

1. Enos, WF, Mann, GT, Dolan, WD: A laboratory procedure for the identification of semen. Am J Clin Pathol 39:316–320, 1963

2. Helpern, M, Wiener, AS: Grouping of semen in cases of rape. Fertil Steril 12:551–553, 1961

3. McCubbin, JH, Scott, DE: Management of alleged sexual assault. Texas Med 69:59–64, 1973

4. Rupp, JC: Sperm survival and prostatic acid phosphatase activity in victims of sexual assault. J Forensic Sci 14:177–183, 1969

ACOG TECHNICAL BULLETIN

NUMBER 14 — JULY, 1970
(Revised, April, 1972)
SUSPECTED RAPE

SUSPECTED RAPE

1. PURPOSE

The purpose of this Technical Bulletin is to provide proper procedures for protection of patient and doctor as well as in the interest of justice in cases of alleged or suspected rape or sexual molestation.

2. DEFINITIONS

Rape is coitus without the consent of the woman.

Statutory Rape is coitus with a female below the age of consent. This is usually 16 but differs in the various States or Provinces.

Sexual Molestation is non-coital sexual contact without consent.

3. CONSENT

To protect the physician, written and witnessed consent for the following procedures should be obtained if possible:

a. Examination

b. Collection of specimens

c. Photographs

d. Release of information to proper authorities.

4. CAUTIONS

The physician must protect the interests of the patient, of justice and of himself. Every instance is a potential court case, and the physician should expect to be subpoenaed to justify his statements. Whether rape occurred is a legal matter for court decision and is NOT a medical diagnosis.

Principal cautions are as follows:

a. GET CONSENT

b. GET HISTORY IN PATIENT'S WORDS

c. RECORD EXAMINATION FINDINGS

d. GET LABORATORY WORK

e. SAVE CLOTHING

f. MAKE NO DIAGNOSIS

g. NOTIFY POLICE

h. PROTECT AGAINST DISEASE, PREGNANCY AND PSYCHIC TRAUMA

5. HISTORY

A good history must be obtained and written down as quotations in the patient's words. The time, place and circumstances should be recorded. The patient's emotional state should also be noted (e.g. hysterical, alcoholic, stoic). Has the patient taken a bath since the alleged assault?

6. EXAMINATION

Get consent to examine from responsible person. Is it legal in your jurisdiction to examine the presumed victim before she has been seen by a police surgeon or similar official? Often the evidence needed to establish guilt or innocence in a case of suspected rape has been thoughtlessly destroyed by a well-intentioned physician.

a. General appearance: bruises, lacerations, torn or bloody clothing and condition of patient (e.g. alcoholic, hysterical, punch-drunk) should be recorded.

b. External genitalia: evidence of trauma.

c. Speculum examination: inspect cervix and vagina with a non-lubricated, but water-moistened speculum. Vaginoscope may be useful.

7. LABORATORY SPECIMENS

The following specimens SHOULD be taken:

a. SWAB from vaginal pool, and from any suspicious areas about the vulva. Protect in test tube. These can be examined by police laboratory for:

(1) acid phosphatase

(2) blood group antigen of semen

(3) precipitin tests against human sperm and blood

b. WET MOUNT of material from fornix examined immediately for motile sperm.

c. Separate SMEARS from vulva.

d. CULTURE for Neisseria in appropriate medium such as Thayer-Martin.

Laboratory specimens should be obtained by a responsible physician in the presence of a witness, and personally handed to the pathologist or technician. They should not be sent to the laboratory by routine messenger service. Unless specimens can be positively identified, the prosecuting attorney may have difficulty in submitting the reports in evidence. Clearly label slides by etching the patient's name on them, using a diamond pencil.

The use of diagnostic tablets will aid in the immediate diagnosis of the presence of acid phosphatase, indicating semen.

8. CLOTHING AND PHOTOGRAPHS

Stained clothing, photographs and any other potential evidence should be retained by the physician and personally turned over to the proper police authorities in return for a detailed receipt.

9. OBJECTIVE STATEMENTS

The record should contain the patient's statements. It should give descriptions of the physician's findings and what he did. It should state to WHOM he delivered specimens, clothing or photographs. The physician should express NO conclusions, opinions or diagnoses to the patient or others. NO conclusions, opinions or diagnoses should be written in the record.

NEVER say or write in the record an opinion concerning whether or not the patient was raped. The phrases "suspected raped" or "alleged rape" may be used when necessary.

The physician should remember that both he and the record may be subpoenaed and that he may be required to testify. All information should be exact and detailed to avoid any misinterpretation. Negative findings are as important as positive ones and may assist in the protection of an alleged assailant who has been falsely accused.

10. CARE OF A CHILD

The protection of a child is an important duty of the physician. Psychosexual trauma must be recognized and minimized. Emotional support and gentle sympathetic understanding of both child and family are very important. The physician must be tactful and kind. The parents should be given reassurance and guidance. They should be warned specifically against magnifying the situation. They should be told to avoid such terms as "ruined," "violated," "dirty," or "lost her innocence" lest the child develop severe guilt feelings and anxiety. It has been shown by many psychiatrists that the child's emotional reaction to sexual molestation is far less damaging than that arising from imposition of adult values upon the episode.

Lacerations should be repaired under general anesthesia. Fine catgut should be used and care taken not to reduce the the size of the introitus. Tetanus toxoid may be indicated inasmuch as these wounds may contain dirt particles and may become infected.

11. PREVENTION OF DISEASE

The attacker may have a venereal disease. For this reason, with the written consent of the family, some physicians customarily give prophylactic antibiotic therapy. In the absence of a penicillin allergy the patient may be given 2.4 million units of benzathine penicillin G (Bicillin®) or an appropriate dose based on age.

12. PREVENTION OF PREGNANCY

The possibility of pregnancy should always be considered. Should exposure occur near midcycle, the administration of large doses of estrogen within 5 days appears to be effective in preventing implantation.

Widest experience has been with diethylstilbestrol 25 mg twice daily, or 50 mg of stilbestrol diphosphate (Stilphosterol®) once daily, for 5 days. Success has also been reported with ethinyl estradiol 5 mg daily for 5 days. The only significant side effect appears to be nausea which occurs in approximately half the patients. This can be lessened with concomitant prochlorperazine (Compazine®) 15 mg spansules once or twice a day.

(continued on back page)

To assist in obtaining the necessary authorizations and data a standardized form is of great value. On the page opposite is a suggested SUSPECTED RAPE form. It may be reproduced or adapted.

MEDICAL REPORT Suspected Rape	 _____ (Hospital Name) Receiving Ward	Date
		Brought by:

Name of Patient	Birthdate
Address	Age

AUTHORIZATION FOR RELEASE OF INFORMATION

I hereby authorize _____ to supply copies of ALL medical reports includ-
(Hospital Name)
ing any laboratory reports, immediately upon completion, to the Police Dept. and the Office of the District Attorney having jurisdiction.

Person
Examined_____

Address_____

Date_____

Parent or
Guardian_____

Witness_____

Address_____

MEDICAL REPORT	Time arrived	Date & Time of Alleged Rape

History (as related to physician)

EXAMINATION	Date	Time

General Examination (include ALL signs of external evidence of trauma)

Laboratory Specimens Collected	**Pelvic Examination** (include ALL signs of trauma, size, and development of female sex organs)
☐ Yes ☐ No (Mandatory, or explain absence)	
	Vulva
	Hymen
Date_____ Time_____	Vagina
Smears ____Vulva ____Vagina ____Cervix	Cervix
	Fundus
Saline Washings ____Vulva ____Vagina	Adnexa (right)
	Adnexa (left)
	Rectal
(Laboratory Reports Attached)	Examining Physician

I hereby certify that this is a true and correct copy of the official_____
Records concerning the examination of the above named patient.   (Hospital Name)

Date   Title

12. Prevention of Pregnancy (Contd.)

Less nausea is encountered if intravenous Premarin® 25 mg a day for 3 days is used, but experience with this method is considerably less than with stilbestrol.

As estrogens are more properly post-ovulatory than post-coital contraceptives, patients should be carefully questioned about prior exposures in the cycle and warned to avoid subsequent unprotected exposures in the same cycle. A basal temperature chart may be useful in determining whether the patient has ovulated. Temperature will usually decline while on estrogen. If the patient does not have a period within 3-4 weeks of treatment, a D&C should be done.

If a pregnancy occurs as a result of rape, its interruption is indicated.

13. FOLLOW-UP OF PATIENT

All patients should be followed to be certain that they do not develop a venereal disease, or become pregnant. The possibility of delayed psychologic effects on child and parents must be remembered. The family physician or a trusted pediatrician is best suited for patient follow-up. In an institutional milieu, one physician should accept the responsibility for supervision and guidance.

14. LOCAL LAWS AND REGULATIONS

The physician must familiarize himself with local laws, regulations and customs. The requirements for police notification vary. If the patient alleges rape, there is usually a duty to report immediately. If rape is suspected, but not stated, "an authorization for release of information" should be obtained.

In some states a physician may not examine a patient until she has been examined by a police surgeon or other authorized medical personnel.

If the child is less than 18 years of age there may be a duty to make an immediate verbal report to designated officials under the "battered child laws."

This Technical Bulletin is prepared (with consultation from appropriate experts) by the Committee on Technical Bulletins of The American College of Obstetricians and Gynecologists. It describes methods and techniques of clinical practice that are currently acceptable and used by recognized authorities. However, it does not represent official policy or recommendations of The American College of Obstetricians and Gynecologists. Its publication should not be construed as excluding other acceptable methods of handling similar problems.

**THE AMERICAN COLLEGE OF
OBSTETRICIANS AND GYNECOLOGISTS**
One East Wacker Drive   Chicago, Illinois 60601

Printed in U.S.A. 9/73

Chapter XIV
ABORTION

Russell S. Fisher, M.D.
Chief Medical Examiner
State of Maryland
Baltimore, Maryland

Definitions

Abortion: Interruption of pregnancy at any time after conception up to the period of fetal viability (usually about the 28th week although occasionally infants born of shorter gestation have survived).

Spontaneous abortion: Occurs without interference from any external agency apparently in 20 to 30 percent of all conceptions; most frequently occurs because of imperfections in the fetus, although maternal abnormalities such as disease of the kidney, uterus, etc. may also be the cause.

Therapeutic abortion: Performed by a licensed practitioner of medicine in order to save the life or protect the health of the pregnant woman in accordance with the laws of the jurisdiction where it is done. Usually performed in a hospital where consultation establishes the indications, surgical records of the procedure are kept, and pathologic examination of the products of conception is made.

Elective abortion: The Supreme Court has ruled that abortion may be obtained at the wish of the pregnant woman. Legal limitations and established customs vary and should be considered in evaluation of such cases, especially where there is a complication which requires official investigation by an agency of the government *i.e.,* police, coroner, medical examiner, district attorney, or public prosecutor, etc.

Criminal abortion: Technically an illegal or extralegal abortion whether self-induced or induced by another. In practice it is of consequence only when attempted, aided, or produced by a second party.

Abortifacient: Any drug or chemical which taken internally or used locally will cause an abortion.

The Investigation of a Death Suspected to be Due to Criminal Abortion

Accidental traumatic vs. induced: Pregnant women are frequently involved in accidental falls, auto accidents, etc. If abortion occurs soon after, the question arises of the role of the trauma in causing it. This is

100

especially so when there is negligence on the part of a second party involved in the accident and civil litigation must be anticipated.

Generally accepted medical opinion holds that accidental traumatic abortions are rare occurrences when there is no serious injury to the mother. Criteria usually regarded as necessary to prove accidental abortion in the absence of severe maternal injury are: (1) the course of the pregnancy preceding the accident must have been normal; (2) pathologic examination of the abortus (fetus and membranes) must not reveal any evidence of abnormal development; and (3) the time interval between the alleged injury and the onset of bleeding or other signs of inevitable abortion must be in minutes or a very few hours at most.[1]

Therapeutic vs. criminal: A therapeutic abortion is an interruption of pregnancy performed to safeguard the health or save the life of the mother. This definition requires that the abortion be performed by a physician acting in the honest belief that the life or health of the pregnant woman will be endangered by continuance of the pregnancy. The more common medical indications for therapeutic abortion are the presence of mental illness or threat thereof, or severe cardiovascular, or renal disease in the mother. Most courts have held that a physician is entitled to the presumption of correct judgment and that he acts in good faith, *i.e.,* if a physician procures an abortion, the state must prove that the abortion was not therapeutic. Physicians have, on the other hand, established by common practices certain minimum evidence of good faith, the absence of which justifies serious doubt of the integrity of the "therapeutic intent." These practices are: (1) the abortion should have been performed by a reputable physician in consultation with a specialist; (2) the physician should have obtained written permission from the husband or guardian as well as from the patient herself; and (3) the operation should have been performed in a reputable hospital and suitable records made of history, physical examination, operation, and results of the pathologic examination of the surgical specimens. Abortion clinics have been established in many States. The procedures used in these clinics have been streamlined, but the principles remain intact.

Methods by which Abortion may be Induced: Therapeutic or elective abortions are ordinarily induced by injections of hypertonic saline into the amniotic sac, or by dilatation of the cervix and curettage of the uterine content. Dilatation of cervix followed by suction evacuation of the uterine contents is a more recently employed variant of the more medically traditional "D and C."

Details of the technics used by criminal abortionists have been well discussed elsewhere.

---

[1] Editors note: At times, the bleeding may be occult, beginning in the potential space between the placenta and the uterine wall. Thus the "interval" between injury and the appearance of the signs and symptoms may be more than just a "very few hours."

101

The incidence of criminal abortion has declined remarkably in recent years since elective abortions have become widely available. During the mid-century decade, it has been estimated that 300,000 criminal abortions per year were performed in the United States. The associated mortality was estimated at 8,000 per year; it is doubtful that it is 800 per year throughout the United States today. This is due to the availability of the much safer elective abortion procedures.

Notwithstanding the marked decrease in criminal abortions in this decade, occasional deaths do occur. The essential proof required to convict an abortionist in instances of maternal death from criminal abortion may be listed in four steps: (1) At the time of alleged criminal act, the dead woman must be proved to have been pregnant. This does not universally obtain and in some States it is immaterial whether or not the woman was actually pregnant. (2) It must be proved that the accused was responsible for the act intending to, or resulting in, interruption of pregnancy. (3) It must be proved that the accused acted for the purpose of producing an illegal abortion. (4) It must be proved that the death occurred as the result of the attempt to interrupt pregnancy.

Source of evidence: The strongest evidence is that given by the eye witnesses, and in non-fatal abortion cases it is rarely possible to gain a conviction without such evidence. Usually only the abortionist and the woman are present when the act is committed. If the woman dies, the abortionist, the only surviving witness, is not likely to provide self-incriminating evidence.

Important evidence may be obtained at the scene where the woman dies, during or immediately after an abortion in the abortionist's office. In these instances the operation may not have been completed and it may be possible to recover some of the remains of the fetus or placenta. If a speciment is recovered it should be transmitted immediately to a pathologist. He can later testify in court, identifying the specimen as a product of recent pregnancy.[2] Photographs of the scene should be taken before disturbance of the premises. Search should be made for instruments that may have been used, soiled clothes, douche apparatus, abortifacient jellies, medications, and the like, all of which should be preserved.

A dying declaration made by the victim of an abortionist can sometimes be acquired in cases when death results from hemorrhage or infection. Such a dying declaration is a statement, made about the cause and circumstances of a homicide, by the victim under the conviction that she is about to die and cannot recover. The statement may be used as evidence in a criminal trial; it is not admissible if the patient recovers. If a physician is the only person available, he should be responsible for

---

[2] Editors note: Immunohematologic technics may be usefully employed here. Absolute proof of the origin of the specimen from the pregnant woman may not be possible to obtain. However, exclusion may be possible and of importance.

recording the statement. In well regulated communities the police are notified of the impending death, so that an officer may be available as a witness to the statement. In obtaining a dying declaration incident to a death from abortion, specific statements should be made to include the following: (1) the dying woman was pregnant; (2) arrangements were made between her and the accused (abortionist) for the purpose of illegally terminating her pregnancy and witnesses who may have been present should be mentioned; (3) an abortion or an attempted abortion did in fact take place, mentioning time, place, and method, insofar as possible; (4) there was or was not bleeding from the vagina immediately prior to the time she submitted herself to the abortionist for operation; and (5) a summary of events following the abortion.

Postmortem examination by a competent pathologist is always essential to provide proof that death did result from causes consistent with the allegation that there was an attempt to interrupt the pregnancy. The pathologist may furnish information, as follows: (1) that the woman had been pregnant; (2) that a criminal abortion had been performed; and (3) that death was the result of the criminal abortion.

Special Procedures

1. Carefully examine the vagina and cervix for injuries made by instruments of abortion.
2. Swabs of the cervix and uterine cavity should be submitted for bacteriologic culture.
3. A blood culture should always be taken.

Do's and Dont's

1. Do investigate thoroughly the sequence of events that preceded the death of a pregnant woman: duration of pregnancy, medical condition of the pregnant woman, marital state, socioeconomic factors, etc.
2. Do visit the scene to look for evidence not usually recognized by inexperienced police officers (*i.e.,* empty ampules, pills, abortifacients, etc.)
3. Do perform a careful autopsy. When death occurs within a short period of time following the procedure, look especially carefully for: air embolism, hemorrhage, foreign body embolisms (*e.g.,* mustard and soap); when death occurs several days after the procedure, infection (with or without hemorrhage) and gas gangrene must be considered.

References

1. Bates, JE, Zawadzki, ES: Criminal Abortion. Charles C Thomas, Springfield, 1964, 250 pp
2. Fisher, RS: Criminal abortion. J Crim Law Criminol, 42:242–259, 1951
3. Newbardt, S, Schulman, H: Techniques of Abortion. Little, Brown and Company, Boston, 1972, 172 pp
4. Schwartz, RH: Septic Abortion. JB Lippincott, Philadelphia, 1968, 153 pp

Chapter XV
FIRE VICTIMS

John F. Edland, M.D.
Monroe County Medical Examiner
Rochester, New York

Introduction

When bodies are recovered from fires the investigation of the cause and manner of death requires the closest cooperation between medical examiner, forensic pathologist, and law enforcement agencies. In most cases it is impossible for the physicians involved to come to any conclusion as to the cause and manner of death without help from those who are investigating the fire just as it is impossible in many cases for the police to arrive at solutions without help from the medical investigator. Unless the forensic pathologist has as many of the facts as can be uncovered concerning what happened prior to the beginning of the fire, his findings are often insufficient to account either for the cause or manner of death.

Scene Visitation

It is important for the medical investigator to visit the scene of the fire in every case. He should not begin his observations until such time as the law enforcement agency and arson investigators with jurisdiction have had an opportunity to make permanent records including photographs and sketches. They in turn should not interfere with the scene until the medical investigator has had time to observe it.

Before the autopsy is begun, every effort should be made to obtain all pertinent information relative to the cause of the fire, the identity of the deceased, if possible, his movements for the preceding few hours, his personality and habits, the names of any witnesses and their statements, etc.

The difficulty of determining the cause and manner of death of a body recovered from a fire will parallel the degree of destruction produced by the fire. The body recovered from a fire generating considerable smoke and not too much heat may be fairly well preserved and the death a result of inhaling hot and noxious gases. The other extreme is a body so completely destroyed that it cannot be recognized as human. This latter situation is, however, most unusual; in almost every case, sufficient material will be available so that certain conclusions can be drawn.

The pathologist presented with a body recovered from a fire is handed several problems. These may include: (1) identification; (2) cause of death and (3) manner of death (*i.e.,* accident, suicide, or homicide).

After a fire, the question frequently arises, "Are the remains human?" This usually can be answered by radiographic examination of the entire remains. The recognition of human bones and teeth, which resist incineration better than other parts of the body is a fairly easy matter. Also, depending on the amount of bony structure remaining, it is often relatively easy from the x-ray film to get some idea of the sex, age, and general build of the individual. On occasion in the debris the remains of a belt or a buckle, safety pins, hair pins, buttons, zippers, etc., will be found which will give a clue to the sex and perhaps the identity of the person involved. If any of the bony structure can be recovered, such as any of the long bones, the spine, etc., fairly satisfactory estimates of height and sometimes even weight can be made. The determination of the race is often a difficult problem; unless there is a fairly complete skull remaining, this is quite often impossible. The teeth must be examined extremely carefully because in many cases this will be the only method by which identification can be made.[1] All articles of clothing and personal objects, such as shoes, belts, key rings, keys, etc., should be carefully noted because they may eventually be the clue to the identity.

Although we use the generic term "burned" as all inclusive, it must be recalled that injury to a person caused by exposure to hot liquids or the vapors arising from them is more properly classified as a scald. A burn is an injury to a person caused by exposure to heated substances, flame, or radiant heat. A scald differs from a burn in that there is no charring of the skin or of other tissues, and no singeing of hair, although the amount of injury may be just as severe in scalding as it is in burning.

The severity of injury depends not only upon the degree of heat applied but upon length of exposure so that burns may vary from a slight reddening of the skin to complete charring of the body. Although there are various classifications of burns ranging from one to six or more degrees, in medicolegal practice burns are usually classified as first, second, or third degree. A first degree burn is superficial; only the skin and subcutaneous tissues are injured leaving in many cases no permanent scar, or if there is scarring, no contracture. Second degree burns are more severe; blisters are formed either immediately or within a few hours, and the soft parts underlying the skin are destroyed in a greater or lesser measure. If the skin only is destroyed, a white, shiny

---

[1] Editors note: A forensic odontologist or a cooperative dentist who is interested in forensic odontology can be of great aid in the examination and interpretation of the dental items recovered. He may also be of utmost value in comparing any recovered teeth and prostheses with dental charts and x-rays.

scar is often left without notable contraction. Burns which cause extensive destruction of tissue may lead to very severe cases of contraction and disfigurement. Actual charring may frequently occur in third degree burns. Extensive third degree burns are always fatal. Obviously, most cases of burns coming to the medical examiner's attention are third degree.

Burns produce severe pain and shock because of the extensive injury to the sensory nerves in the skin. Death may occur quickly from immediate shock with vasomotor collapse, or may be delayed a few hours. If the injury is not sufficient to cause death within a few hours, the patient may subsequently succumb to secondary causes such as pneumonia, septicemia, lower nephron nephrosis, etc. If the victim dies shortly after receiving burns, the internal abnormality found at autopsy will be non-specific, consisting mostly of congestion of the viscera.

The external examination of the body is of special importance in every case of death due to burns. The radiographic examination (referred to previously) for the purpose of identification can be used, of course, to reveal the presence of foreign bodies (e.g., bullets) or other injuries (e.g., fractures). The blisters observed on any recognizable epithelium should be carefully examined as blisters formed as the result of postmortem putrefaction differ from the blisters of antemortem burns by the absence of an inflammatory reaction and by the elevation of the entire epidermis from the corium to form the covering of the blister. Blisters produced by heat usually have a high content of albumin in the blister fluid and, of course, there may be an inflammatory reaction about the blister.[2] On examining the body externally, one should note the presence or absence of any fractures, but it should be recalled that fractures may be produced by sudden contraction of the muscles. In severe third degree burns of the body, the muscles are so contracted as to produce a typical posture known as the "pugilistic attitude." This resembles the appearance of a person trying to defend himself in the classical manner of the boxer.

The intensity of the heat may produce long splits in the skin, occasionally resembling lacerations and more rarely, incised wounds. In many cases where the body is burned while lying on a hard surface, the portion adjacent to the hard surface may be remarkably intact. The body should be examined closely for odors of petroleum products or other flammables.[3]

After a careful external examination, the body should be opened in the usual manner and a thorough examination of the internal organs

---

[2] Editors note: The presence or absence of an inflammatory reaction will depend upon how long the burn was present prior to death. A minimum of two or more hours will be necessary under usual conditions.

[3] Editors note: Even in instances where no odor of an inflammable (incendiary) substance can be detected, such substances may be detected by distillation of remnants of clothing from the body.

made. Forensic pathologists are familiar with the fact that although extensive external charring of the body may be present, often there is surprisingly little injury to the internal organs. When one recalls the high water content of the body this is not difficult to understand.

Once the body is opened, particular attention should be given to the color of the viscera as many persons who die accidentally during a conflagration die not as the result of burns but as the result of inhalation of noxious gases, notably carbon monoxide. When the body is opened, a sample of blood should be withdrawn and sent to the laboratory for determination of the amount of carbon monoxide (carboxyhemoglobin) in the blood. A small amount of carbon monoxide is normal but levels higher than 10 percent are not.[4] Levels in excess of 45 percent are lethal and indicate that the individual died as a direct result of the fire (carbon monoxide asphyxiation). If blood cannot be obtained from the heart, every effort should be made to obtain it elsewhere. Only a small quantity of blood is required, and it may even be necessary to saw a long bone in two and extract cells from the bone marrow. Whenever possible blood should be taken to determine if alcohol is present in the blood, and for other toxicologic and chemical examinations.

All organs of the neck and chest, including the tongue, are then removed en bloc. The glottis, epiglottis and trachea, and large and small bronchi are examined carefully for evidence of the effects of heat and inhalation of hot gases. This may consist of reddening, blistering, and actual destruction of the wall of the trachea and large and small bronchi. One should also carefully look for the presence of particulate matter of a carbonized nature (smoke) which has been inhaled during the course of the fire. The presence of any pathologic changes or the presence of these materials is good evidence that the person was alive when the fire began. Its absence does not, of course, necessarily mean that the person was dead when the fire started. However, the absence of any carbon monoxide in the blood of a person found dead in a burned house would be strong presumptive evidence that the person was dead when the fire began, as this type of fire is invariably accompanied by a large amount of smoke which usually asphyxiates the victims.

The internal organs should be carefully examined for evidence of trauma or natural disease which might have produced death prior to the fire. The hyoid, the thyroid cartilage, the soft tissues of the neck, etc., should be carefully examined to rule out strangulation. A full description of any pathologic changes in the internal organs should be given, and the absence of any organs as the result of surgical procedures

---

[4] Editors note: Some very heavy smokers may have carboxyhemoglobin levels of 13 to 15 percent; traffic control officers in canyon-like streets in large cities may accumulate up to 20 percent.

should be noted for the latter may be a valuable clue to the identification of the victim. Sufficient material should be retained for microscopic and chemical examinations.

Special attention should be given to the examination of the head because artifacts may be present which can be most misleading. In cases where the flame was in contact with the head and there is extensive charring of the skull, the intense heat may cause a postmortem transudation of blood between the dura and calvarium. This appears as an amorphous brown-red deposit and is usually totally unlike the usual disk-shaped traumatic epidural hemorrhage. This postmortem extradural "hemorrhage" is probably the result of a combination of factors produced by the intense heat which caused a local shrinking of dura and brain and postmortem rupture of vessels on the outside of the dura; during the burning of the body, blood is also forced from the trunk into the head and then into the extradural space through the ruptured vessels. Postmortem fracture of the vault of the skull may occur in connection with the charring and if associated with extradural hemorrhage, can be mistaken for antemortem injuries and erroneously interpreted as evidence of "foul play."

When fractures are present at the base of the skull, one can assume that these are not produced as a result of the "steaming" of the brain. Such fractures, of course, may be the result of secondary injury during or following the fire such as falling beams, etc.

In the event that any evidence of "foul play" is recovered, (such as bullets) the continuity of evidence must be carefully maintained.

The medical examiner and the forensic pathologist also must give their attention to assigning the manner of death. The death, of course, may be due to natural disease processes, accident, suicide, or homicide. As a generalization, in most cases when bodies are recovered from fire scenes, the deaths are of an accidental nature. Suicide by fire is quite rare. Homicide by burning (other than those deaths occurring during an arsonous fire) is exceedingly rare, but burning to destroy evidence of homicide is not uncommon.

On occasion, the assignment of a manner of death may present an extremely difficult problem. For example, in the files of the Chief Medical Examiner (Monroe County, New York) there is a case of a man found dead on his sofa with severe burns of the entire body. The premises had been almost completely gutted by fire. At the autopsy it became evident that the burns had been received after death. Postmortem examination revealed a rupture of the heart through an old scar; investigation by the medical examiner revealed that the deceased had been treated for some time for heart disease, that he was a chain smoker, and that there was no evidence to support anything suspicious. It was surmised that he was lying on his sofa watching television when he

108

suffered his fatal attack. The cigarette he was smoking dropped on the sofa and this caused the subsequent fire.[5]

When there are indications that the individual was dead before the fire started and postmortem evidence of injury by an outside agency (*i.e.,* firearm wounds, stabbing, throttling, etc.) a strong presumption of homicide is raised, and the case should be handled as such until the contrary is proven. An excellent example of this is seen in the case for the Chief Medical Examiner's (Monroe County, New York) files of a 78-year-old man found dead in his apartment above his shoemaker's shop. He was known to smoke in bed and small fires had occurred on previous occasions. There seemed to be little doubt that death occurred as the result of fire caused by smoking in bed. However, postmortem examination revealed the presence of a large defect in the right parietal bone with extensive fractures into the base of the skull and involving the strongest portion, the petrous portion of the temporal bone. Also, a sample of blood with no carbon monoxide present indicated that the decedent was dead before the fire began. Subsequent investigation by the police revealed that the decedent had been robbed and murdered and that the fire was set after death to conceal the crime.

There is a strong suspicion of homicide when death occurs before the fire and there is evidence death was due to violent means other than the fire. When death occurs after the fire and no other cause of death can be assigned other than the fire, there is a strong probability the death was accidental. However, it should be borne in mind that the strength of this probability decreases in direct proportion to the extent of destruction of the body by the fire. The usual signs of death by throttling, suffocation, or blows may be completely destroyed by fire.

In an investigation of deaths of persons recovered from fire, the following points should be emphasized:

1. Following a fire a thorough investigation should be conducted to ascertain the possibility of the presence of unsuspected victims.
2. The circumstances surrounding the fire should be carefully investigated by the medical examiner and law enforcement agencies, such as the police, fire marshals, etc., and all this information should be given to the forensic pathologist prior to the beginning of the autopsy.
3. When the presence of human remains is known or suspected the medical examiner should be notified immediately so that he or his deputy may proceed to the scene.
4. Adequate photographs and sketches of the scene should be made.
5. A thorough, extensive, complete, and unhurried postmortem ex-

---

[5] Editors note: Checking the urine toxicologically for the presence of nicotine would yield evidence that a person was, in all probability, a smoker. Non-smokers do not have detectable levels of nicotine in the urine.

amination should be made by an experienced pathologist having the necessary equipment and physical facilities for such an examination.
6. Finally, the most valuable tool in the investigation of the dead body recovered from a fire is a high index of suspicion and unlimited curiosity in the minds of all those engaged in the investigation.

References

1. Gonzales, TA, Vance, M, Helpern, M, Umberger, CJ: Legal Medicine, Pathology and Toxicology. Second edition. Appleton-Century-Crofts, New York, 1954, pp 250–270
2. Peterson, F, Haines, WS: A Text-book of Legal Medicine and Toxicology. Volume I. WB Saunders, Philadelphia and London, 1903–04, 730 pp
3. Spitz, WU, Fisher, RS: Medicolegal Investigation of Death. Charles C Thomas, Springfield, 1973, 536 pp

Chapter XVI

ELECTRICAL INJURIES AND LIGHTNING

John F. Edland, M.D.
Monroe County Medical Examiner
Rochester, New York

Introduction

Although deaths from lightning and the electric chair are often dramatic, electrical energy involving low tension or low voltage currents commonly employed in the home and industry cause most accidents and death from electrical shock.

Exposure to electricity is universal in life today, and the possibilities of injuries are endless. Industry is unthinkable without electricity. A housewife's self-esteem may depend upon the numerous appliances by which her home overwhelms that of her neighbors. "Do-it-yourself" gadgets expose her husband to electrical dangers. A small child plays at electrical outlets; the young person plays with radio, television, and electric motors. Electricity close to bathtubs establishes high hazard. Quite "unfunny" jokes, sometimes fatal, are played with electric shock. High tension wires cross our landscapes and pose special problems. No direct contact is necessary as a 10,000 volt spark will travel as far as 3.5 centimeters. Static electricity remaining in wires after opening the switches or induced electricity from adjacent lines carrying alternating current may shock and frighten, and may cause fatal accidents by falling. In moist weather even the safest insulation may acquire a wet conducting surface. These facts must be kept in mind if claims are made that injury or death by electrical energy was impossible as "all safety measures" were taken.

The cause of death in electric injuries varies. Low intensity current of 25 to 75 milliamperes causes cardiac arrest during diastole which, if continued for more than 30 seconds, will be followed by fibrillation. Low voltage kills immediately or not at all. Currents from 75 milliamperes to 3 or 4 amperes give rise to cardiac fibrillation and currents of higher intensity to cardiac standstill or arrhythmias. Burns at the point of contact may increase resistance to the current and thus, decrease its intensity. Because of this the less dangerous high intensity current may decrease to a lower tension in which fibrillation is produced instead of the more easily reversible cardiac standstill. Current passing through the respiratory centers of the brain may result in respiratory death. Injuries and burns, rather than the current itself, may cause death.

The autopsy findings in death from lightning are non-specific. According to Strassmann[8], the main findings include: (1) fluid blood in the heart and larger vessels; (2) moist and distended lungs; and (3) congestion of the parenchymatous organs, brain, and meninges with occasional hemorrhages. Some epicardial and subendocardial hemorrhages and subserosal and mucosal hemorrhages of the respiratory and gastrointestinal tracts are found.

The majority of deaths directly due to electrical energy are those involving low tension or low voltage currents used in the home and industry. There are marked differences in the effects of this type of current in the body from those produced by lightning or high voltage currents.

Accurately and technically, the term "low voltage" refers to currents of 1,000 volts or less, but currents of 110 to 220 volts are the primary concern. Before considering the subject in detail, it is necessary to discuss some of the variables other than voltages, some of which are of much more importance and which may determine the results of a given stimulus.

Variables in Electric Shocks

1. **Variations in the current.** The first group of variables is the properties of the current: voltage, amperage, frequency, and direction. Paradoxically, shocks from high voltage electricity are relatively more safe than shocks from lower voltage electricity. Ram[6], in a survey of electrical accidents in England from 1912 to 1921, determined that 63 percent of those receiving a shock greater than 650 volts recovered while only 39 percent of those receiving a shock of less voltage lived. This is due to the selective action of high voltage electricity on the nervous system and respiratory apparatus which permits effective treatment by artificial respiration in many cases. Lower voltage electricity acts on the conduction system of the heart to produce ventricular fibrillation which is frequently fatal.

A more important factor than the voltage is the amperage or amount of current flowing. The high amperage of high tension wires causes them to be extremely lethal; however, it is impossible, after an accident, to estimate accurately the amperage involved as it is dependent upon so many other variables, particularly the resistance. It has been estimated that the maximum current to which a person (between an arm and a leg) may be safely subjected is 0.1 ampere for a duration of one second. As most electrical appliances carry much heavier amperage than this, the danger is apparent.

A third important property of the electrical current is its direction,

112

alternating current being four to five times as dangerous as an equal voltage of direct current. Deaths from contact with direct current of less than 300 volts are rare while contact with 25 volts of alternating current is dangerous if the skin is moist and a large contact is made. An important property of alternating current is the frequency. Muscles and nerves are relatively sensitive to currents of high frequency (greater than 100,000 cycles Hertz) and are especially sensitive to 60 Hertz current in common use.

2. **Variations in the contact.** A second group of variables affecting the mortality from electric shocks is the properties of the contact areas: its resistance, the area involved, the duration of current flow, and the pathway taken by the current in the body.

The resistance varies considerably with grounding, moisture, area of body involved, insulation, etc., all contributing to the variations. The resistance of dry skin is from 900 to 1000 ohms, but the resistance of wet skin is from 200 to 300 ohms. The increase in amperage according to Ohm's law (Amps = Volts/Ohms) would, therefore, be three- to fourfold. Good grounding conversely increases the resistance to current flow and is a great protection.

A critical characteristic of the contacts is the pathway of the current through the body. A current of a very dangerous voltage may cause little or no damage if it passes from a leg to the ground, whereas a current of relatively safe voltage may cause a fatal arrhythmia if it passes from the head through the electrical field of the heart and out a lower extremity.

The area of a contact is a third important feature as well-placed electrodes will lead to far less resistance and, therefore, increased current flow with correspondingly greater consequences (*e.g.,* an electrocution or shock causing a tetanic grasp of a live wire).

The duration of the contact is an important component of electric shock as the more prolonged the contact, the more likely that fibrillation will occur.

External Evidence of Injury

One of the difficulties encountered in investigation of deaths by electrocution with currents of low voltage is that there may be absolutely no evidence of any injury either on the clothing or on the body. In many instances, the injury will be confined solely to the clothing. Thorough external inspection of the body is an absolute must. The clothing, including shoes, gloves, and head gear should also be carefully examined. This is especially true in electrical injuries because there may be burns on the outside as well as on the inside of garments without injury to the skin. Marks from passage of the current are not always found; occasionally, only the hair is singed. Helpern and Strassman[2] found marks in only one-third of all electrical accidents observed in which the tension was 220 volts or less; however, they were found in all cases involving as much as 600 volts and higher.

The appearance of current marks varies. They are generally depressed, firm, glistening areas which may be pale, or yellow, brown, black, or greenish due to carbonization of material from the conductor. The area surrounding the marks is frequently raised from contraction and peripheral edema. Erythema may be present. The shape of the mark often corresponds to that of the contact surface. Sometimes the current travels along the surface or may even jump and enter at some distance from the point of contact. Direct current may cause, on the negative pole, swelling only. High amperage has an explosive effect and may produce injuries resembling bullet, stab, or cut wounds. Small balls of molten metal, derived from the metal of the contacting electrode, so-called current pearls, may be carried deep into the tissue.* If the clothing catches fire during an electrical injury, as often happens with high tension wires, it may be difficult or even impossible to discover current marks on the clothing or the burned skin.

Current marks may be hidden inside the oral cavity where they occur from putting live wires into the mouth, as children do, or from drinking at a water fountain in contact with electric current. Similarly they have been found in the urethra as a result of voiding on a high tension wire (example: a child voiding from a trestle over an electric railroad line). Urine, because of its high content of electrolytes is a good conductor.

A special type of electrical injury is caused by lightning. When a body is found dead in the field, the investigating officer may not think of lightning as the cause of death. The typical lesion from lightning is an arborescent dendritic or leaf-like figure on the skin due to vascular dilatation with or without hemorrhages. Burns may appear as zigzag lines. Lightning marks may simulate gunshot-like perforations of the skin, or dried out spots of bird droppings. As in other electrical injuries, the body surface may not present any evidence and only the inside of the clothing exhibit burns. If blisters are formed, they are more likely due to electrolytically formed gas than to burns. Microscopically, lightning marks show no palisading of the nuclei. Hemorrhages in the skin are often most pronounced about the hair papillae. Metal objects carried by the victims often become magnetic and this characteristic can be used to establish the possible cause of death.

---

* Editors note: Analysis of this material for elemental content may yield identification of the offending electrode. Elemental comparison of the suspected electrode with the "pearl" may establish without doubt the actual electrode involved. A reverse analysis, using hair, skin, blood group substance analysis and comparison may also yield results of high confidence in establishing the nature of the electrode and the point of contact with the victim.

The diagnosis of electrical injury by autopsy depends on finding a current mark which may be represented only by a small burn either on the clothing or on the body, and if it is not present, on history and knowledge of the circumstances and the absence of other causes of death. Electrocution or lightning is often not suspected when the body is "submitted" for autopsy without accompanying information as to the circumstances of death.

Autopsy Findings

Rigor mortis often sets in early. Hemorrhages in the conjunctivae are common. The electrical current follows the routes of least resistance, which are the blood filled vessels, and thus may reach the heart even though it does not lie in a straight line between entrance and exit. The heart tends to stop in diastole and is generally dilated, especially on the right side. Epicardial and subendocardial hemorrhages are often present. As in other types of sudden death, the blood is frequently fluid. There may be necrosis of the intima or of the complete wall of blood vessels. The elastica interna may split from the wall. Thromboses may occur, especially in arteries. Capillaries may rupture due to the sudden rise of blood pressure from tetanic contractions; thus, hemorrhages occur. The lungs may be congested or edematous, or both, especially when death is due to damage of the respiratory center. In extensive burns, the fatal outcome may be due to hemoglobinuric nephrosis. Skeletal muscles in the path of the current may show Zenker's degeneration, often with spiraling and fragmentation of the fibers. Bones and joints may be damaged by trauma or from a fall or from tetanic contractions; or heat generated by the current may melt the calcium phosphate into bony "pearls." There may be hemorrhages in the brain, especially in the ventricles. Thromboses occur in the meninges and edema in the cerebral substance. Heat may even cook the brain. A fetus may survive the electrocuted mother, or a surviving mother may abort after electric injury.

Late sequelae of electrical injuries are important from an insurance standpoint. Angina pectoris can occur immediately or a few days after an injury. It may disappear or myocardial necrosis may lead to a delayed death. Thromboses can lead to edema and gangrene of limbs. Permanent damage to the spinal cord with multiple sclerosis and amyotrophic lateral sclerotic-like symptoms have been described. Cataract and cloudiness of the cornea may appear many years after the electrical injury.

As in all medicolegal problems when the postmortem findings are nonspecific, the following is essential: (1) that the forensic pathologist have full knowledge of the details surrounding the death and access to the scene if necessary; (2) that the autopsy be conducted in a proper area having adequate lighting and equipment; (3) that extensive care be taken in examining the clothes and the external appearance of the

115

victim; and (4) that the examining forensic pathologist have a high index of suspicion.†

References

1. Bennet, IL: Electrical Injuries, Principles of Internal Medicine. Third edition. Edited by TR Harrison, McGraw-Hill Book Company, New York, 1958, pp 802–804

2. Helpern, M, Strassmann, G: Circumstances and postmortem findings, especially skin lesions, in accidental electrocution. Am J Pathol, 17:592–594, 1941

3. Lerokove, E, Morris, MH: Auricular fibrillation after electric shock with complete recovery, case report. New York J Med, 54:807–808, 1954

4. Lewis, GK: Trauma resulting from electricity. J Internat Coll Surg, 28:724–738, 1957

5. MacFarland, D: Electric shock: cause, incidence, and consequences. Arch Phys Ther, 18:99–102, 1937

6. Ram, S, with Legge, TM, Levy, AG, and MacWilliam, JA: The pathological changes produced in those rendered insensible by electric shock and the treatment of such cases. Arch Radiol Electrotherapy, 27:112, 1922

7. Spitz, WU, Fisher, RS: Medico-Legal Investigation of Death. Charles C. Thomas, Springfield, Illinois, 1973, pp 311–321

8. Strassman, G: Effect of heat and low temperature, electric current and radiation, Legal Medicine. First edition. Edited by RBH Gradwohl. CV Mosby, St. Louis, 1954, pp 195–219

9. Strauss, AF, Mann, GT: Forensic pathology seminar. J Forensic Sci, 5:184–191, 1960

10. Wehrmacher, WH: Atrial fibrillation due to accidental electric shock. JAMA, 165:349–351, 1957

---

† Editors note: The examination of the appliance that was in use at the time of death may be an important link in establishing death as being due to the effects of electrical energy. The services of an electrical engineer may be of invaluable help. The use of commonly available low-cost devices to determine the presence or absence of adequate grounding of the duplex outlet into which the appliance was plugged, may establish the break in electrical safety responsible for the electrical energy injury or death.

Chapter XVII
HEAT AND COLD

Michael M. Baden, M.D.
Deputy Chief Medical Examiner
New York, New York

Introduction

Accurate diagnosis of death due to extremes of environmental temperature is dependent on a complete knowledge of the circumstances of death. Autopsy findings are nonspecific.

Heat stroke (sun stroke) refers to a rapid increase in body temperature with a dry hot skin. Body temperatures are often found to be above 106° F and have been recorded above 112° F. This is always associated with high environmental temperature (above 90° F) and high humidity. This is an uncommon and serious condition. The rise in body temperature is due to inability of the body to lose heat by evaporation of sweat. Death results from peripheral circulatory failure. Other common but much less serious hyperthermic disorders include heat cramps and heat exhaustion. These are due to excessive loss of sodium and chloride in sweat. Heat stroke occurs most often during the first few days of a heat wave. It is often associated with physical exertion and frequently occurs in alcoholics and in persons with chronic illnesses.

Prolonged exposure to cold can result in body temperatures below 90° F. Cardiac arrhythmias and shock frequently follow. Fatalities due to exposure to cold most frequently occur among alcoholics who fall asleep outdoors in freezing weather. Localized cold injury (frostbite and immersion foot) can lead to extensive gangrene.

Preliminary Steps

1. Obtain complete information regarding the circumstances of death, including initial body temperature if available.
2. Be aware of the local environmental temperature and humidity during the previous few days.

Autopsy

1. Autopsy findings in heat stroke are subtle and include degeneration of neurons in the cerebral cortex, cerebellum and basal ganglia, and scattered petechiae in the walls of the third and fourth ventricles

288-953 O - 79 - 9

and the aqueduct. Petechiae also may be found in the thoracic and abdominal viscera. Postmortem decomposition begins early and progresses rapidly. Localized application of heat to the skin can result in burns of varying degrees (see Chapter XV). Death resulting from cold and exposure is associated with bright red postmortem lividity. Cutis anserina (goose-flesh) may be present because of rigor of the arrectores pilorum muscles. The onset of decomposition is delayed, and the process is slowed. Postmortem freezing of a body, regardless of the cause of death, may cause ice to develop in body fluids and fractures of cranial bones, especially along suture lines. Fatty liver or cirrhosis and pneumonia are frequent findings at autopsy, not because of their specificity of relationship with cold, but because they frequently mirror the lifestyle of the individual who does as a result of exposure.

Do's and Don'ts

1. Do consider the possibility of heat stroke in all unexplained deaths during hot weather. Occasionally body temperatures of 108° F or greater will be caused by intracranial disorders which can be excluded at autopsy.[1]
2. Do measure the body temperature at the scene of death or soon thereafter before the body is refrigerated. Determination of the rectal temperature may be made at the scene; temperature of the liver can be determined as soon as the body is opened, or by means of a small incision over the liver area upon arrival of the body at the morgue.
3. The environmental temperature is, of course, of great importance. The weather bureau can supply data regarding temperature, humidity, wind velocity, cloud cover, etc. All of these data must be interpreted with regard to the environment where the body was exposed. Temperature, air movement, radiant heat bodies, moisture, etc. must be noted at the scene.
4. Do determine the level of alcohol in appropriate body fluids or tissues.
5. Do consider the possibility of homicide in deaths results from exposure to cold.

References

1. Malamud, N, Haymaker, W, Custer, RP: Heat stroke. Military Surgeon 99:397–449, 1946
2. Talbott, JH: The physiologic and therapeutic effects of hypothermia. New Engl J Med 224:281–288, 1941

[1] Editors note: During hot summer weather there is a rapid rise in temperature in the passenger compartment and trunk of automobiles left exposed to the sun. This rapid temperature rise may easily cause the death of small children and animals left unattended in the automobile while the parent shops.

Chapter XVIII
THE NECK

Leslie I. Lukash, M.D.
Chief Medical Examiner
Nassau County, New York

Charles S. Hirsch, M.D.
Associate Pathologist and Deputy Coroner
Cuyahoga County Coroner's Office
Cleveland, Ohio

Introduction

1. All too often, the neck is the "no man's land" of the autopsy. This is unfortunate because competent and skillful examination of this area is absolutely essential in medicolegal autopsies. Injuries inflicted by cutting, stabbing, and firearms are omitted from the discussion which follows.

2. The presence or absence of externally visible cutaneous injuries and their appearance are determined by the amount of force applied, rate and duration of application of force, and the surface area involved in energy transfer.

   a. The more rapidly a force is applied, the more likely it is to produce injury (*e.g.,* sudden squeezing of the neck in contrast to gradual compression).

   b. The smaller the area of application of force, the more likely it is to produce nonuniform, injurious displacement of tissues (*e.g.,* narrow ligatures are more likely to produce abrasions than are broad ones; fingernails are more likely to produce abrasions than are forearms).

   c. The longer a compressing ligature remains on the neck, the more likely it is to produce a permanent furrow.

3. **Hanging** usually leaves an inclined furrow on the neck which duplicates the size and pattern of the rope (electrical cord, belt, etc.) if the individual was suspended for a prolonged interval. Victims who are discovered promptly and "cut down" may have no cutaneous furrow. Ordinarily the furrow is situated above the level of the thyroid cartilage, rises to a suspension point at the occiput or posterior

119

aspect of the neck, and has its low point 180 degrees opposite the suspension point.

The cause of death by hanging, in most instances, is compression of the cervical vasculature and not asphyxia by airway obstruction. If this compression halts venous return from the head for an appreciable interval prior to cessation of arterial flow to the head, it causes intense venous engorgement above the level of the ligature with petechiae of the eyelids and conjuctivae. When arterial flow is obstructed rapidly by the compressing force, the former findings are absent and death results from cerebral ischemia.

Internal injuries of the neck are uncommon in hanging. Characteristically there is minimal or no hemorrhage in the cervical soft tissues, and fractures of the laryngeal cartilages or hyoid bone do not occur in a typical hanging. Fracture of the rostral cervical vertebral column is the "objective" of a judicial hanging and occurs only as a result of a properly placed noose and a drop of sufficient length (based upon body weight) to cause fracture but not decapitation.

Many hangings are accomplished from suspension points below the individual's standing height (*e.g.,* door knob).

4. **Ligature strangulation.** The external stigmata produced by ligature strangulation are determined by the same variables enumerated above. The most important distinctions from a hanging furrow are that the mark of a ligature strangulation is oriented horizontally on the neck, does not rise to a suspension point, and usually is situated below the level of the thyroid cartilage.

Internal cervical injury resulting from ligature strangulation is variable. In the majority of instances, it is more severe than that caused by hanging and less severe than that produced by manual strangulation (see below).

In rare instances, individuals accomplish suicide by ligature strangulation. This requires that the ligature be knotted or otherwise fastened so that cervical compression is maintained following loss of consciousness. It follows that manual self-strangulation is impossible.

5. **Manual strangulation.** Manual strangulation typically is characterized by the presence of small contusions and abrasions in groups on the front and back of the neck. Patterned, crescentic abrasions duplicating the assailant's fingernails are classical. The assailant need not have long fingernails to inflict such injuries. Petechiae of the eyelids and conjunctivae are frequently, but not invariably present.

Internal cervical hemorrhage is the rule in manual strangulation, and fractures of the hyoid bone or laryngeal cartilages, or both, are common. However, there may be no fractures, particularly when the victim is young and has considerable elasticity of the latter structures.

120

6. Compression of the neck by a smooth surfaced, broad object (*e.g.,* forearm) may leave no external or internal injury.
7. Extreme injury of the internal cervical structures (*e.g.,* bilateral comminuted fractures of the larynx) usually is caused by a blow to the neck or a fall on the neck rather than manual strangulation. In these situations, the fractured margins are driven inward (hinged toward the outside), whereas in manual strangulation squeezing of the sides of the hyoid bone and larynx causes the fractured margins to point outward (hinged toward the inside).
8. **Internal airway obstruction**
   a. Fatal aspiration of a bolus of food needs explanation. It is rare for a neurologically intact, sober individual with natural teeth (adult or child) to die by aspirating a bolus of food. By contrast, terminal or agonal aspiration of liquid and finely particulate gastric content is common and has absolutely no pathologic significance unless the individual lives long enough to develop aspiration pneumonia.
   b. Fatal aspiration of foreign bodies (nuts, coins, balloons, etc.) occurs in children.
   c. Suppurative epiglottitis (almost invariably due to *H. influenzae,* type B) causes an occasional childhood fatality and sometimes occurs in adults.
   d. Anaphylatic fatalities (bee stings, penicillin, etc.) usually show obstructive edema of the arytenoepiglottic folds (not the vocal cords).
9. Injuries of the cervical vertebral column and spinal cord are frequently missed. The neck organs should be removed, the anterior longitudinal ligament of the vertebral column exposed and examined, the posterior aspect of the neck incised and dissected down to the spinous processes, and the ligaments surrounding the rim of the foramen magnum and odontoid process incised.

Preliminary Steps

1. Photograph injuries.
2. If a ligature is present on the neck (hanging or strangulation), photograph it prior to removal, and remove by cutting away from the knot so that it can be easily reconstructed.

Autopsy

1. Dissect the neck organs after the thoracic viscera and brain have been removed. This will decompress the cervical veins and help to minimize artifactual hemorrhage.
2. It is helpful to have an assistant who can hold a pair of small or medium-size surgical rake retractors.
3. Use only sharp dissection; never cut blindly.
4. Following removal of the neck organs, examine the areas of the

common carotid artery bifurcations for hemorrhage. Examine the vertebral column as mentioned previously.

Pitfalls and Pearls

1. The female victim of strangulation or cervical compression should be examined for evidence of rape (see Chapter XIII). Strangulation implies rape until proven otherwise.
2. Insects (*e.g.,* ants, roaches) can denude the skin in a fashion strikingly similar to fingernail abrasions.
3. Beware of misinterpreting creases on the neck of an infant or resuscitation trauma as stigmata of ligature strangulation or smothering (see Chapters XI, XII).
4. Absence of externally visible neck injury does not preclude the possibility of underlying fatal trauma.
5. Absence of internal cervical hemorrhage in a hanging victim does not mean that he was suspended post mortem.
6. A diagnosis of death by cervical compression (in the absence of external and internal injuries) requires a detailed history and a complete autopsy (including indicated toxicologic studies) to exclude other causes of death.
7. Aspiration of gastric content is a much used and abused diagnosis. Do not confuse terminal aspiration of regurgitated food with a pathologically significant event.
8. See Chapter XXI for a discussion of hangings related to sexual practices.

References

1. Lachman, E: Anatomy of judicial hanging. Resident and Staff Physician, 18(7):46–54, 1972
2. Teeters, NK, Hedblom, JH: Hang by the Neck. Charles C Thomas, Springfield, 1967, 483 pp

Chapter XIX
ASPHYXIAL DEATHS

Allan B. McNie, M.D.
Forensic Pathologist
Alameda County, California
Oakland, California

Introduction, Concepts, and Principles
1. **Mechanics of respiration.**
   a. Central stimulas, may be depressed by drugs
   b. Rib action, increases both AP and the transverse diameters
   c. Diaphragm descent
   d. Lung expansion
      (1) The pleural surfaces are held in apposition by a fluid layer, "lungs follow chest wall."
      (2) Potential negative pressure may be obliterated (*i.e.,* pneumothorax)
   e. Alveolar-capillary exchange may be impaired as in carbon monoxide deaths
2. **Definition.** Asphyxiation is the end stage of significant interference with the exchange of oxygen and carbon dioxide.
3. **Classification of mechanisms of asphyxia.**
   a. **Traumatic asphyxia** is external compression of chest. Traumatic asphyxia is more frequently seen in infants and young children, and in adults in industrial accidents, or in victims of automobile crashes.
   b. **Suffocation is obstruction** at mouth and nose. Suffocation is seen as a cause of death in infants (*i.e.,* accidental death from a plastic bag) or as a form of homicide (*i.e.,* an individual under the influence of alcohol or other drugs) or deliberate suffocation of an infant. Suicide with a plastic bag is occasionally seen.
   c. **Obstruction in mouth or pharynx.** This mechanism of asphyxia is seen in:
      (1) **gagging,** seen most often in homicides
      (2) **positional asphyxia,** where the weight of the body produces forcible flexion of the neck on the chest
      (3) **postictal respiratory failure** is the mechanism in epileptics where the togue falls against the posterior pharyngeal wall

123

d. **External compression of the neck.**
   (1) **Hanging** (where the weight of the body tightens the ligature) is frequently seen. Body need not be completely suspended, is rarely homicidal, but is occasionally accidental (see Chapter XXI, Adolescent Sex Hangings).
   (2) **Manual strangulation** (where an arm or hands constrict the airway) is invariably homicidal.
   (3) **Ligature strangulation** is where an external force tightens the ligature.
e. **Obstruction of larynx.**
   (1) **Foreign body obstruction,** occurs most frequently in drunks, the aged, and children and is often overlooked.
   (2) **Laryngeal edema,** may be caused by allergic or anaphylactic reactions, infections, tumors, or as a result of an irritant gas.
   (3) **Laryngospasm,** no anatomic evidence. It is a diagnosis of inference and exclusion (suspicion must be present that such a mechanism exists).
f. Obstruction within *tracheobronchial* tree.
   (1) Drownings[1]
   (2) Aspiration, most frequently of gastric contents but may also be seen in blunt injuries, hemorrhage and aspiration of blood.
g. Interference with *gaseous exchange.*
   (1) carbon monoxide poisoning
   (2) oxygen pneumonopathy
   (3) cyanide (interference at cellular level)
   (4) anoxic environment as occurs in an industrial setting, hydrogen sulfide, carbon dioxide, etc.

4. **Signs of asphyxiation.**
   a. General signs. These are not pathognomonic nor are they invariable and each can be seen in other conditions unrelated to asphyxiation.
      (1) **Cyanosis,** is most apparent above the site of obstruction.
      (2) **Petechial hemorrhages.** These occur most frequently on the conjunctivae, eyelids, face, galea aponeurotica, and serosal surfaces. Several mechanisms are operative such as anoxic alteration of capillary permeability and increased intravascular pressure.
      (3) **Postmortem fluidity of blood.** Is frequently seen and may clot after removal from body.
      (4) Congestion and edema of the lungs are frequently seen.

---

[1] Editors note: Drowning with death due to asphyxia occurs in only 10 to 20 percent of cases of submersion.

(5) There may be dilatation of the right sided chambers of the heart and petechial hemorrhages in the myocardium.

(6) There may be congestion, swelling, or petechial hemorrhages in the nervous system.

b. Specific signs.

(1) **Traumatic asphyxia.** Injuries, contusions or abrasions, are frequently seen at point of compression. Rib fractures may be seen. Petechial hemorrhages seen above point of compression. Face may be "black" from suffused blood in some accidents. This mechanism is sometimes seen in victims of motor vehicle crashes.

(2) **Suffocation.** There may be small or faintly discernible contusions or lacerations on inner aspects of lips. Petechial hemorrhages may be seen. Look for cloth fibers in injuries about mouth. Suffocation from a plastic bag is seen more frequently in the elderly than in infants, and adults are usually under influence of sedative drugs or alcohol.

(3) **Gagging.** Tongue is forced against palate and there are usually injuries to the mouth. The gag is frequently held in place by a ligature which causes grooves or contusions at the lateral angles of the mouth. Intense cyanosis and petechiae are frequently seen. In some cases the ligature may have been removed before the body was discovered (same applies to bindings).

5. **Positional and postictal respiratory failure.** A history of epilepsy and a documentation of body position are crucial in diagnosing these cases. Often only the general findings of asphyxia are present.

Drowning. (See Chapter XX)

6. **Hanging.** Encircling groove usually cants upward toward one ear or toward the occiput (toward point of suspension). Abrasions from the knot are often seen near an ear. Groove is above laryngeal prominence, shows erythema at the edges, and often displays pattern of ligature. Injuries to soft tissues of neck may be minimal. Conjunctival petechial hemorrhages are rarely seen. Laryngeal cartilages and bones are rarely fractured. Cyanosis is often intense. Protrusion of tongue and gravitational stasis are present.

7. **Manual strangulation.** External evidence of strangulation may be obvious with fingernail marks, contusions, and abrasions, or may be completely absent. Fractures of laryngeal cartilages and bones are very frequently found, most commonly of the cornua or thyroid cartilage, the hyoid bone, and the cricoid cartilage. In infants and children there may be no fractures. Hemorrhage should be associated with fractures. Careful dissection of the neck with avoidance of artifacts is mandatory. Petechial hemorrhages are plentiful.

125

Occasionally there are no fractures, only submucosal hemorrhages of the larynx.[2]

8. **Ligature strangulation.** Encircling ligature (or groove) usually is not canted and there is damage to structures immediately beneath ligature. Intense cyanosis and petechiae are seen above the ligature. In women, rape should not be ruled out.

9. **Foreign body obstruction.**
   a. Is very frequently overlooked. One death in 800 is due to foreign body obstruction of airway.
   b. Cases are recognized by:
      (1) Doing a complete autopsy
      (2) All people who die in likely situations such as kitchens, rest homes, bars, and restaurants should be autopsied.
   c. External signs of asphyxia are non-existent
   d. Consider the possibility that a foreign body was removed or dislodged during resuscitative attempts.

10. **Laryngeal edema**
    a. Amount of edema will decrease with the postmortem interval. Only wrinkling of mucous membrane may be present.
    b. Eosinophiles may be seen microscopically.
    c. Drug antibodies may be demonstrated.

Preliminary Steps

1. **Examination of undisturbed scene.**
   a. Is extremely important.
   b. Photographs may be used to supplement investigative information.

2. **Take photographs.**
   a. for identification
   b. to document wounds
   c. to show knots and bindings

3. **Gather trace evidence.**
   a. Use a hand-lens or dissecting microscope
   b. Look for fibers about mouth and nose
   c. Clip the fingernails
   d. Examine for rape which is frequently observed in female victims of strangulation
   e. Remove bindings or trussing by cutting and taping to board. Do not untie or disturb knots.
   f. Collect samples of hair
   g. Know the anatomy of the neck

---

[2] Editors note: Manual strangulation without either "external" or "internal" evidence is very rare, but can take place.

Autopsy

1. **Perform a complete autopsy** in every instance.
2. **Neck dissection**
   a. Adequate exposure is mandatory
   b. Dissect by muscle layers
   c. Examine the ligaments
   d. Dissect tissue from the larynx to expose any fractures
   e. Examine tongue
   f. Expose the spinal column
   g. Document positive and pertinent negative findings
   h. Do not rush dissection
3. **Take tissues** for microscopic examination.
4. **Collect samples.**
   a. Blood for ABO, MN grouping (and possibly other blood group analysis) alcohol, and sedatives
   b. Smears of vagina, mouth, and anus as indicated
   c. Specimens of liver and urine (save by freezing)
   d. Samples of scalp and pubic hair from homicide cases
5. **Autopsy** all persons who die while eating, who are found dead with food nearby, or who die in rest rooms at meal time regardless of history of pre-existing disease.

Special Procedures

1. **Trace evidence** may be of vital importance. Look for it and protect.
2. Take **proper specimens** to ascertain if rape occurred.
3. **Preserve bindings** or rope-ties; do not untie.
4. Order **x-rays** which may be helpful to document injuries.
5. Open vessels in neck **longitudinally** to show intimal laceration.
6. **Asphyxial deaths** from exclusion of oxygen
   a. are usually industrial
   b. tie off the trachea and use a vacutainer to obtain a sample of air from within the trachea, or place entire lung in a sealed container
7. **Drownings.**
   a. Obtain differential chlorides
   b. Look for hemorrhage in the middle ears
   c. Importance of the demonstration of diatoms in tissues is questionable.
8. **Fingernail scrappings.**

Do's and Don'ts

1. Do have all history available prior to beginning postmortem examination
2. Do preserve evidence—do not destroy it

3. Do provide adequate exposure in dissection of the neck and do not produce iatrogenic fractures
4. Do recognize how frequently signs of asphyxia are seen in people who die suddenly from heart disease. (The most commonly encountered cause of petechial hemorrhages in the conjunctivae is "pseudo-strangulation" syndrome.)
5. Do examine all cases for drugs, particularly alcohol and sedatives
6. Do consider other causes of fractures
   a. Blunt injuries
   b. Clothes line injury
7. Do consider artifact from tight collar
8. Do not mistake articulations for fractures; look for possible accompanying hemorrhage.
9. Do not consider signs of asphyxia as absolute
   a. Not all signs are present in asphyxial deaths
   b. Some signs of asphyxiation may be present in non-asphyxial deaths
10. Do not stop short of a complete autopsy
11. Do not mistake evidence of resuscitation for signs of strangulation
    a. Holding head for resuscitation
    b. Incubation injuries

References

1. Modell, JH: Drowning and Near-drowning. Charles C Thomas, Springfield, 1971, 119 pp
2. Polson, CJ: The Essentials of Forensic Medicine. Charles C Thomas, Springfield, 1965, pp 286–401

Chapter XX
DROWNING

William G. Eckert, M.D.
Deputy Coroner, Sedgwick County
Wichita, Kansas

Charles S. Hirsch, M.D.
Associate Pathologist and Deputy Coroner
Cuyahoga County
Cleveland, Ohio

Introduction

Drowning is death due to submersion in a fluid, any fluid. For practical purposes, we are concerned only with drowning in water, because drownings in other fluids are uncommon, frequently bizarre, occurrences which are evaluated and interpreted by the same principles as are water drownings.

Most drownings are accidents; however, some persons intent upon suicide choose drowning as their method, frequently in conjunction with jumping from a bridge or other high place. Homicidal drowning is a suspicion generally aroused by finding a body submerged in a bathtub.

Death by drowning is a diagnosis made on the basis of history, circumstances surrounding death, and a complete autopsy (including toxicologic studies) to *exclude* other possible causes of death.

There is no objective, morphologic finding which is pathognomonic of drowning.

The so-called "drowning tests" (all of them, including demonstration of diatoms) are not diagnostic of drowning when positive, and do not exclude a diagnosis of drowning when negative.

Pathophysiology. In fresh water drowning, aspirated water (hypotonic fluid) is absorbed rapidly across pulmonary alveolar capillaries. This causes acute expansion of blood volume, hemolysis, and hemodilution with resulting cardiac arrhythmias and failure.

The reverse of the foregoing occurs in seawater drowning. Seawater is approximately 3 to 4 percent sodium chloride; when this hypertonic fluid is aspirated, it draws water from the capillaries into alveoli causing pulmonary edema.

129

Preliminary Steps

Familiarize yourself with all available information concerning the circumstances surrounding death.

If the decedent is clothed, make note of the type and condition of clothing; preserve it.

Photograph injuries.

Autopsy

Anatomic findings in drowned victims are nonspecific. They may include pulmonary congestion and edema with white or blood-tinged froth in the nose,[1] mouth, and distal respiratory passages; hemorrhage in the middle ears (remove the dura mater from the floor of the skull); water in the stomach and air passages; and aspiration of gastric content. A small proportion of drowned individuals will have nonedematous ("dry") lungs.

Negative findings are as important as the positive. Drowning is a diagnosis by exclusion and the autopsy must rule out injuries and disease as contributory or alternative causes of death. Therefore, the autopsy of a drowned victim must be complete, and should include toxicologic studies.

Incapacitating or fatal trauma to the head or neck may occur without externally visible injury. Competent evaluation of the cervical vertebral column may require incision of the posterior aspect of the neck, incision of the ligaments surrounding the odontoid process and at the margins of the foramen magnum, and inspection of the anterior longitudinal spinal ligament following removal of the neck organs.

If samples are to be saved for a "drowning test," obtain blood from the left and right sides of the heart using separate dry syringes and needles and place the samples in appropriately labelled containers.

Water Artifacts. Decomposition and putrefaction proceed at a rate determined primarily by temperature. Cold water preserves bodies; warm water hastens putrefaction.

Adipocere, a soap-like transformation of subcutaneous tissues, forms on bodies submerged for prolonged intervals (months), but may be present in as little as six weeks time.

Fish and other marine animals gnaw exposed parts of submerged bodies in a fashion similar to postmortem mutilation by rats, mice, or carnivorous house pets.

Boat propeller injuries usually are multiple, smoothly marginated wounds in a parallel arrangement.

Postmortem abrasions and lacerations of the skin can be extensive. Such injuries result from scraping the bottom or battering against solid objects. The typical pattern of abrasions from scraping the bottom is

---

[1] Editors note: This is seen in pulmonary edema from any cause—*e.g.,* drug overdose, congestive heart failure, and severe head injuries.

distributed over prominent points on the face and anterior surface of the trunk and extremities because submerged bodies assume a face down attitude unless trapped by debris or vegetation. However, battering by waves can produce an infinite array of injuries. Distinction between antemortem and postmortem injuries can be extremely difficult. Antemortem injuries should be associated with hemorrhage into soft tissues, adjacent to fracture sites, or within body cavities. Remember not to be dogmatic when in doubt.

Bathtubs. People die in bathtubs for the same reasons they die in bed or elsewhere in the home. It is untenable to conclude that anybody but a small child has drowned in a bathtub unless disease (*e.g.,* epilepsy), intoxication, or injury renders him helpless in such an unfortunate situation.

Interstitial pulmonary emphysema, pneumothorax, and air embolism may be seen when death has occurred during scuba and deepsea diving. When dealing with such diving deaths examination of the equipment is essential; do not tamper with it unless you have the requisite expertise to evaluate it properly.

Pitfalls and Pearls

Beware of the neck. Do not fail to remove the neck organs and look for vertebral fractures.

Aspiration of gastric contents occurs commonly during the unconscious gasping phase of drowning. It is a result of, and not the cause of, drowning.

Include phenobarbital and Dilantin in your toxicologic survey on drowned individuals. The presence of therapeutic quantities of these drugs may be the single clue that the deceased person was suffering from epilepsy; absence or very low levels of the drugs in a known epileptic may help to explain the drowning.

Do not rely on a "drowning test" either to make or exclude a determination of drowning.

Water and aquatic debris in the stomach and lungs are not diagnostic of drowning. Bodies submerged after death can show similar material in a similar distribution.

A few hundred milliliters of putrefactive fluid frequently accumulates in each pleural cavity in decomposing bodies and is not indicative of either drowning or injury.

References

1. Eckert, WG: Drowning in 40 year indexed compilation of the International literature, 605 references. Inform, 1971
2. Eckert, WG: Diving and underwater problems in 40 year indexed compilation of the International literature, 895 references. Inform, 1971.
3. Eckert, WG: Dangerous marine animals and foods in 40 year indexed compilation of the International literature, 803 references. Inform, 1971

4. Miles, S: Underwater Medicine. Third edition. JB Lippincott Co, Philadelphia, 1969, 363 pp

5. Model, JH: The Pathophysiology and Treatment of Drowning and Near-Drowning. Charles C Thomas, Springfield, 1971, 119 pp

Chapter XXI
ADOLESCENT SEX HANGINGS

John F. Burton, M.D.
Chief Medical Examiner of Oakland County
Pontiac, Michigan

Introduction

Cause of Death: Asphyxia due to hanging.

Manner of Death: Accident.

Motive. Sexual gratification through masturbation.

Sex Aberration: Auto-erotic sadomasochism.

Definition: Self generated sexual activity directed toward one's self, aided by self infliction of injury and being recipient of mistreatment for sexual gratification.

Diagnostic Features

1. Certain features at the scene confirm the act. (Do not disturb, cut down or alter anything until the following is documented by photographs).
2. The scene of death is usually a locked bathroom or some part of the home not frequently trespassed such as the attic, basement, or utility room.
3. The victim is usually a nude or partially nude male between 12 and 20 years of age.
4. He is found hanging by the neck, supported by a towel or rope covered by a towel, loosely wrapped around the front of the neck in such a manner that trauma is unlikely and removal is easy.
5. The head is tilted forward and the face downward. The hands, occasionally bound loosely at the wrists, are free to touch the genitals. Occasionally the victim wears the clothing of the opposite sex (transvestism).[1]

---

[1] Editors note: Not really "transvestism," as the person usually does not expose himself to others dressed in clothing of the opposite sex. Most frequently, the clothing consists of panties, bra, sanitary belt, stockings, etc.

6. The legs are usually bent at the knees, with the feet touching the floor but bearing no weight at the time the body is found.
7. There may be semen in the urethral meatus or on the floor beneath the hanging victim. A positive smear is helpful in confirming the circumstances of the act.[2]
8. Photographs of the scene "as is" are mandatory before the body is cut down because afterwards, "it becomes just another hanging."

Autopsy Findings

1. A furrow in the skin on the front and sides of the neck caused by the towel or rope used to suspend the body which was so loosely applied about the neck that its pressure could have been released by hand or by merely standing erect.
2. Deep lividity is present in the skin of the face and neck, above the ligature; petechial hemorrhages are present beneath the conjuctivae; bloody mucus may be present in the nares and mouth due to extravasation from the mucus membranes of the nasopharynx and oral cavity; and at times bits of vomitus are present.
3. Visceral changes include dark red fluid blood in the cardiac chambers and acute passive congestion of all organs.
4. As the autopsy findings do not differ from those of hangings in general, the sex, age, and circumstances at the scene are all important to the pathologist in classifying the death.

Incidence

The incidence is rare. Although the number of persons who practice this type of activity are numerous, the existence of such is known only by the fatal cases that are discovered at wide intervals of time. Such deaths occur more frequently in the large cities of the United States. In many instances these deaths are veiled in secrecy and ignorance, and in some parts of the country they are still regarded as suicides. The age of the victim is usually 12 to 20 years and rarely over 40. The sex is predominantly male, although, rarely, females have been reported. The etiology is unknown. The source of this idea is interesting and has been a favorite question of many students of the subject. Some suspected points of origin are: (1) person-to-person communication; (2) pornography; (3) French novels; (4) soldiers who served in the China-Burman-India war theatre; (5) Oriental sex practices; and (6) last but not least, "instinctive experimentation."

Concept

Although auto-erotic sadomasochistic death during masturbation is regarded as an accident by consensus, different theories exist about the circumstances leading to death. There are some who believe that the

---

[2] Editors note: Ejaculation during hanging is not rare and may occur without masturbation.

134

practitioners of this activity are aware of the possibility of death as evidenced by the precautions taken in preparing for the act. This group theorizes that during the ecstasy the victim loses consciousness and becomes helpless to release himself, the trance-like state results in a fatal cerebral anoxia and the hanging causes death.

Others believe that although sexual gratification was expected and death was unintentional, the interim course of events changed when the victim, intent upon climax, misjudges the existent anoxia already present and time required to reach orgasm by masturbation. There is also the additional consideration that at the particular moment, the victim really does not care about his safety.[3]

---

[3] Editors note: Investigation of death which is caused by hanging to intensify masturbatory sexual gratification is of great importance to different people and groups. The parents or wife or husband may be convinced that the act was of a suicidal nature. The law enforcement groups may suspect murder. For the proper settlement of insurance, the accidental manner of death is important and might be successfully challenged if documentation of the case is weak.

Chapter XXII

CHARACTERISTICS OF WOUNDS PRODUCED BY HANDGUNS AND RIFLES

Frank P. Cleveland, M.D.
Coroner, County of Hamilton
Cincinnati, Ohio

Introduction, Concepts, and Principles

1. **Class and individual characteristics of bullets and cartridge cases.** To understand the principles used in the identification of firearms it is necessary to know what takes place when a cartridge is fired.

    a. **Class characteristics.** When a cartridge is fired, it separates into two major components: a casing and a bullet. When a weapon is manufactured, a predetermined number of grooves (rifling) are cut into the bore of the firearm. This causes the bullet to spin and to assume a gyroscopic action which stabilizes the bullet in flight. The rifling may have a right or left twist. The number of grooves, direction of twist, and caliber make up the so-called class characteristics of the firearm.

    b. **Individual characteristics.** When the rifling is cut into the barrel, the tools used to cut the grooves in the bore leave individual markings due to chattering, chipping or wear. These markings vary from one finished barrel to the next barrel produced and are, therefore, individual and distinctive in each. When a cartridge case is struck by the firing pin, the firing pin also may produce distinctive markings upon the base which are reproducible. As the pressure from expanding gases forces the bullet forward into the barrel, the cartridge case is pushed back against the breech face or recoil plate. The force of this impact transfers marks left by milling to the cartridge case and these markings are reproduced on each cartridge fired in the same firearm. When an extractor pulls a discharged cartridge from the chamber, it, too, may leave distinctive markings, and when the ejector throws the discharged cartridge from the weapon, this also may transfer distinctive markings to the cartridge case. (Table I)

2. **Mechanism of injury.** The magnitude of physical injury depends upon the quantity of energy possessed by the projectile (and transmitted

136

to the target). This is determined by the velocity and the mass of the bullet.

The translational [1] kinetic energy of a bullet expressed in ft-lbs equals one-half of the product of its *mass* expressed in slugs and its velocity in ft/sec squared. This is expressed as $KE = \dfrac{1}{2} mv^2$.

A slug is the mass possessed by an object weighing 32 pounds. The weight of bullets is designated in grains with 7,000 grains equal to 1 pound. Therefore,

$$KE = \frac{1}{2} \frac{\text{wt in grains}}{1} \times \frac{1\ lb}{7{,}000\ \text{grains}} \times \frac{1\ \text{slug}}{32\ lbs} \times \frac{v^2\ \text{in ft/sec}}{1}\ \text{or}$$

$$KE = \frac{1}{2} \frac{\text{wt in grains}}{7{,}000 \times 32} \times v^2\ (\text{in ft/sec})$$

Example 1: KE of a .38 Special 158 grain bullet at 800 ft/sec.

$$KE = \frac{1}{2} \frac{158}{7{,}000 \times 32} \times (800)^2 = 225\ \text{ft-lbs}$$

Example 2: KE of a .30–06 rifle bullet of 150 grains at 3,000 ft/sec.

$$KE = \frac{1}{2} \frac{150}{7{,}000 \times 32} \times (3{,}000)^2 = 3{,}000\ \text{ft-lbs}.$$

Thus, increasing velocity by 3.75-fold or 375 percent produced a 1,333 percent or 13.333-fold increase.

Preliminary Steps

1. **Preservation of evidence.**
   a. **Protect the clothing.** Remove carefully, examine, label, and store for further examination. Air dry if wet.
   b. **Protect the body.** Do not wash or cleanse until samples have been taken for examination for powder residues.
   c. **Protect the hands.** Cover with plastic bags [2] so that examination may be made as indicated below.

2. **Nature of ancillary examinations available.**
   a. **Technic for detection of trace metals.** Contact between metal and skin produces a reaction which becomes visible with ultraviolet light when the chemical 8-hydroxyquinoline is applied.
   b. **Paraffin glove technic.** Hot paraffin applied to skin will dislodge powder residue which then may be detected by applying diphen-

---

[1] Editor's note: This does not include the rotational energy possessed by the bullet as a result of spinning.

[2] Editor's note: Sweating may occur when the body is refrigerated prior to removel of plastic bags. Ordinary paper bags may cause less skin maceration.

TABLE I. *Characteristics of guns.*

Ways and Means of Identification	Revolvers	Auto-Loading Pistols	Rifles	Shotguns	Homemade Guns and Zip Guns
Lands and grooves	Yes; most common, 4 to 10, right or left twist	Yes; most common 4 to 12, right or left twist	Yes; 2 to 22, right or left twist	None	No; most zip gun barrels made from automobile antennas or length of pipe
Bullets	Class and individual striae	Class and individual striae	Class and individual striae	Size of shot or rifled slug	Presence of rifling marks on bullet
Discharged cartridge casings	Firing pin indentation; recoil plate mill marks	Firing pin indentation; breechface or mill marks; ejector and extractor	Firing pin indentation; breechface marks; ejector and extractor	Firing pin indentation; breechface marks; extractor and ejector; wadding	Firing pin marks
Powders	Flake, granule, ball; few black still in use	Flake, granule, ball; few black	Flake, granule, ball, stick; few black	Flake, granule, ball, few black	Flake, granule, ball
Type of Bullets	Most common of all lead or half-jacketed; sometimes full jacketed	Almost always full-jacketed	.22 cal short, long or long rifle: lead; center fire; most always metal jacketed	Rifled slug (largest) to size #12 shot	Most are .22 cal but can be made to shoot rifle, pistol or revolver ammunition

ylamine reagent to the paraffin glove. A blue color reveals the presence of fine particles of nitrate.[3]

c. **Neutron activation analysis.**[4] Residue from primer can be removed from hands by wiping with swabs moistened with 5 percent nitric acid. The swabs are irradiated and the radioactive primer particles can be identified and quantitated using radioactive counting technics.

Examination of Wounds

Wounds from revolvers, pistols, and rifles will have characteristics which vary depending on the velocity of the bullet (which is the largest factor determining the destructive energy).

1. **Classification of wounds.**
   a. **Abrading or grazing wound.** Marginal abrasion of the skin along a central shallow furrow.
   b. **Lacerating wound.** Laceration or tearing of the cutaneous surface surrounding the entrance defect. (A special type is the stellate entrance wound described below.)
   c. **Penetrating wound.** A bullet wound where there is only an entrance and no exit.
   d. **Perforating wound.** A wound characterized by both an entrance wound and an exit wound.
   e. **Wounds from high velocity projectiles.** Increasing the velocity of projectiles increases geometrically the quantity of energy produced and this produces perforating wounds with unusual features: bone may literally be pulverized; soft tissue laceration may be widespread and at considerable distance from the track of the projectile; lacerations may be observed within the intima of arteries; exit wounds may be unusually large.

2. **Characteristics of typical wounds.**
   a. **Entrance, tight contact.**
      (1) On the body surface
         (a) Central defect
         (b) Marginal abrasion (contact ring) of uniform width
         (c) Powder residue deep in wound
         (d) Gaseous residue distributed internally with separation along fascial planes
         (e) Peripheral abrasion from gun barrel and sight around contact ring

---

[3] Editor's note: This classic "paraffin test" is non-specific and has been abandoned by many in favor of other technics.

[4] Editor's note: A similar technic for collection of primer residue can be utilized and analyses carried out by atomic absorption technics. It is also a useful and sensitive technic.

    (2) In the skull
        (a) Stellate lacerations radiating from the central defect
        (b) Marginal abrasions (contact ring), powder residue deep in the wound
        (c) Gaseous residue distributed along fascial planes
        (d) May be internal explosive fractures of skull
        (e) Bone fragments become secondary missiles
        (f) Peripheral abrasions around contact ring from barrel and sight

b. **Entrance, loose contact**
    (1) Central defect
    (2) Marginal abrasion (contact ring)
    (3) Powder residue upon the skin surface and within the track of the wound.

c. **Entrance, close.**
    (1) Central defect
    (2) Marginal abrasion (contact ring)
    (3) Cutaneous tattooing or stippling from particulate powder and metallic residue

d. **Entrance, distant.**
    (1) Central defect
    (2) Marginal abrasion (contact ring)

e. **Entrance, atypical.**
    (1) Irregular, elongated entrance defect caused by instability or tumbling of bullet and the physical character of the tissue involved
    (2) Irregular abraded margins
    (3) Lacerations of cutaneous tissue

f. **Exit wound.**
    (1) Lacerated irregular defect with everted margins and sub-cutaneous fat protrusion.
    (2) May be larger than entrance wound, secondary to deformity of bullet or secondary missiles (*i.e.,* bone).[5]

g. **Interpretation of marginal abrasion** (contact ring).
    (1) Bullet acts like drill rotating against skin while stretching skin beyond its limit of elasticity
    (2) When bullet is perpendicular to surface, contact ring is of relatively uniform width
    (3) When bullet is at a tangent to the surface, contact ring is of an irregular width and widest border indicates directional relationship of bullet to target.

---

[5] Editor's note: Exit wounds in areas where the skin is supported by clothing, etc. may not resemble the usual outshoot wound. In such instances, the defects may be circular and the margin may appear abraded. Such wounds are sometimes termed "shored" outshoot wounds.

Example: Direction

Perpendicular   At an Angle

h. **Note:** "Tight contact wounds" and "distant wounds" may have similar external characteristics and can only be distinguished after dissection.

i. **Characteristics of bone defects produced by bullets perforating the skull.**

   (1) The entrance wound in bone has a punched out appearance in the internal table and has a larger, beveled defect in the internal table.

Example:

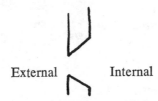

External   Internal

   (2) The exit wound in bone has a punched out appearance in the internal table and has a larger, beveled defect in the outer table (the reverse of the entrance defect).

Example:

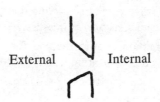

External   Internal

3. **Description of wounds.**

   a. **Describe the external characteristics of entrance wounds.** Specify the size of the defect and the width of the contact ring; locate, using fixed points of the body for reference.

   b. **Describe the course and direction of the bullet(s)** through the body using planes of the body (*i.e.,* horizontal, sagittal, and coronal).

   c. **Describe all organs and tissues through which the projectile passes** and include the size of the defect(s) or lacerations pro-

141

duced; include specific vessels injured and note the quantity and location of internal hemorrhage; note secondary missiles related to fracture of bone.

    d. **Locate and describe characteristics of the exit wound** if projectile perforates the body.

4. **Recovery of evidentiary material.**
   a. **Locate bullet by x-ray, fluoroscopy, or dissection:** remove by careful, fine dissection; do not grasp with metallic instruments (mutilation may result).
   b. **Label projectile on base** with specific and unique identifying mark or symbol. DO NOT MARK ON THE SIDE![6]
   c. **Maintain continuity of possession:** place in labelled container; deliver personally to next person to keep chain of evidence intact; identify, label, seal, sign, and deliver.

5. **Microscopic examination of wounds.**
   a. **Prepare section from wound of entrance** to demonstrate injury and powder residues.
   b. **Prepare section from depth of wound** to demonstrate powder residues.

Special Procedures

1. **Photography of wounds.**
   a. **Black and white photographs.** To demonstrate size, location, and physical characteristics.
   b. **Color photographs.** To demonstrate the same as black and white.
   c. **Infrared photographs.** Excellent technic to demonstrate powder residue on clothing.

2. **X-ray examination.**
   a. To locate bullets.
   b. To demonstrate fragments of metal and bone.
   c. To show course and direction of missiles.

3. **Fluoroscopic examination.** Rapid method for locating bullet or foreign material and for demonstrating fractures of bones.

4. **Chemical reaction.** Swabs, extracts, or tissue samples may be taken for determination of powder residues.

5. See above for analyses for trace metals, powder and primer residues.

Postmortem Examination

Conduct examination according to technic described elsewhere in this manual.

---

[6] Editor's note: One system which might be employed is to mark the base (or nose) of the bullet with the initials of the deceased and a number to specifically identify each bullet, such as, RJ–1, RJ–2, etc. Other systems are easy to devise. The description of bullet markings should be made apart of the autopsy protocol.

Pitfalls and Pearls

1. Do preserve clothing.
   a. For correlation with wounds upon the body.
   b. For examination of defects to determine entrance and exit from examination of the fibers.
2. Do use x-ray and fluoroscopy for location of projectiles or foreign bodies and to aid in their recovery.
3. Do mark projectiles in the proper place for identification purposes.
4. Do recover fragments. They may be necessary for determination of caliber and examination to identify weapon from which projectile(s) was fired.
5. Remember that projectiles may undergo internal richochet after striking bone, especially in the skull.
6. Remember that projectiles may enter blood vessels or spinal canal and be transported great distances from the site of entrance or track of the wound.
7. Do not attempt to predict the caliber of the bullet from the size of the entrance wound.
8. Do not predict that the entrance would is a "distant" wound or a "contact" wound until after the wound has been dissected.
9. Do not produce any alteration or distortion of projectiles by careless dissection.

References

Editor's comment. Many articles (and even books) have been written about firearms injuries. Some of these are out-of-date; others deal with very specialized topics. The following three general references may be of use to the pathologist who has occasion to examine bodies when death was caused by injury from firearms:

Spitz, WU, Fisher, RS: Medicolegal Investigation of Death. Charles C Thomas, Springfield, 1973, 536 pp

Sturner, WQ, Petty, CS: Firearms injuries, Modern Trends in Forensic Medicine 3. Edited by AK Mant. Butterworths, London, 1973, pp. 120–138

Petty, CS: Firearms injury research. Am J Clin Pathol 52:277–288, 1969

Also, two useful references pertain to the histologic examination of gunshot wounds:

Adelson, L: A microscopic study of dermal gunshot wounds. Am J Clin Pathol 35:393–402, 1961

Rolfe, HC, Curle, D, Simmons, D: A histological technique for forensic ballistics. J Forensic Med 18:47–52, 1971

Chapter XXIII
SHOTGUN WOUNDS

Charles S. Hirsch, M.D.
Associate Pathologist and Deputy Coroner
Cuyahoga County Coroner's Office
Cleveland, Ohio

Introduction

Definition of terms and basic concepts

1. **Gauge** refers to the internal diameter of the shotgun barrel (bore) and is expressed in two systems:
   a. Whole numbers. The smaller the number, the greater the diameter of the barrel (*e.g.,* a 10 gauge shotgun has a bore diameter of 0.775 inch; a 20 gauge shotgun has a bore diameter of 0.615 inch).
   b. Decimal fractions. The bore diameter is represented in hundredths of an inch [*e.g.,* .410 ("four ten")].[1]

2. **Choke** refers to internal constrictions of the distal part of the shotgun bore designed to better keep the pellets together in flight. The greater the degree of choke, the smaller is the shot pattern at a given range. (Tables I and II.)
   a. **Cylinder bore** means no choke.
   b. **Full choke** is the highest degree of bore constriction.
   c. Shotguns may have **variable choke** adapters.
   d. Double barrel shotguns may have a different choke in each barrel.

3. **Components of shotgun shells.**
   a. Primer and powder
   b. Wads, which may be:
      (1) Felt or cardboard disks located between the powder and the shot and between the shot and the distal end of the shell. These are called undershot and overshot wads, respectively. The latter are not present in most modern shells;

---

[1] Editors note: In the United States the .410 bore shotgun is the only one commonly available using this system of nomenclature. Some European shotguns are classified by the metric system (*e.g.,* 9 mm.).

144

TABLE I.[2] *Approximate Spread of Shot in Inches at Various Distances.*

	5 Yards	10 Yards	15 Yards	20 Yards
Cylinder	8	20	26	30
Half-choke	5	12	16	20
Full-choke	3	9	12	15

TABLE. II.[2] *Percentage of Shot Falling Within a 30-inch Circle at Various Choke Adjustments.*

Choke Adjustment	Average %
Full-choke	70
Three-quarter choke (improved modified)	65
Half-choke	60
Quarter-choke (modified choke)	55
Improved cylinder	50
True cylinder (no choke)	30–40

instead the distal end of the shell is closed by crimping the casing material ("star crimp").

(2) Plastic cups which contain the shot, either alone and serving as a wad, or in combination with felt wads.

c. Shot or pellets (Table III)

(1) Shot size is expressed by numbers. The smaller the number, the larger the shot (*e.g.,* #12 shot has a diameter of 0.05 inch and #6 shot has a diameter of 0.11 inch).

(2) Buckshot. Again, the smaller the number, the larger the pellets. These are manufactured by two standards of measurement: Eastern size (#4 is the smallest and 000 is the largest) and Western size (#8 to #9 is the smallest and #2 is the largest).[3]

(3) Rifled slugs are single large projectiles loaded in a shotgun shell.

4. **Classification of wounds.** All of the components of shotgun shells may contribute to the wound pattern, depending upon the range of fire. Spread of the shot pattern is determined by range of fire, choke, barrel length, and type of ammunition.

---

[2] Tables I and II are taken from Breitenecker, R: Shotgun wound patterns. Am J Clin Pathol 52:258–269, 1969 and are reprinted here with the permission of the author, Rudiger Breitenecker, M.D., Baltimore, Maryland, the *American Journal of Clinical Pathology,* Dallas, Texas, and the Williams and Wilkins Company, Baltimore, Maryland.

[3] Editors note: The Eastern nomenclature is now standard in the United States. Western nomenclature is rarely encountered.

TABLE 3A. American Shot Sizes.

Shot No.	Diameter (mm.)	Diameter (in.)	Chilled Shot Weight/Pellet (Gm.)	Chilled Shot Weight/Pellet (gr.)	Chilled Shot Approximate No. of Shot/Ounce	Drop (Soft) Shot Weight/Pellet (Gm.)	Drop (Soft) Shot Weight/Pellet (gr.)	Drop (Soft) Shot Approximate No. of Shot/Ounce
Dust	1.02	0.04						4565
12	1.27	0.05	0.0117	0.18	2385	0.0124	0.19	2326
11	1.52	0.06	0.0254	0.32	1380	0.0215	0.33	1346
10	1.78	0.07	0.0325	0.50	868	0.0338	0.52	848
9	2.03	0.08	0.0488	0.75	585	0.0501	0.77	568
8	2.28	0.09	0.0689	1.06	409	0.0715	1.10	399
7½	2.41	0.095	0.0819	1.26	345	0.0859	1.29	388
7	2.54	0.10	0.0939	1.46	299	0.0975	1.50	291
6	2.79	0.11	0.1274	1.96	223	0.1300	2.00	218
5	3.02	0.12	0.1651	2.54	172	0.1790	2.60	168
4	3.30	0.13	0.2084	3.21	136	0.2152	3.31	132
3	3.53	0.14	0.2601	4.01	109	0.2678	4.12	106
2	3.78	0.15	0.3431	4.97	88	0.3302	5.08	86
1	4.06	0.16	0.3894	5.99	73	0.4004	6.16	71
B	4.32	0.17	0.4810	7.40	59			
Air Rifle	4.44	0.175	0.5200	8.00	55			
BB	4.57	0.18	0.5720	8.80	50			
BBB	4.83	0.19	0.6760	10.40	42			
T	5.08	0.20	0.7930	12.20	36			
TT	5.33	0.21	0.9165	14.10	31			
F	5.59	0.22	1.0630	16.20	27			
FF	5.84	0.23	1.1830	18.20	24			

TABLE 3B. *Buckshot*

Eastern Size	Western Size	Diameter In (mm.)	Diameter In (in.)	Approximate No./Lb.	Weight In (Gm.)	Weight In (gr.)
4		6.09	0.24	341	1.333	20.5
3	8–9	6.35	0.25	299	1.528	23.5
2	7	6.86	0.27	238	1.918	29.5
1	5–6	7.62	0.30	175	2.600	40.0
0	4	8.13	0.32	144	3.153	48.5
00	3	8.64	0.34	122	3.738	57.5
000	2	9.14	0.36	103	4.420	68.0

Tables 3A and 3B are taken from Breitenecker, R: Shotgun wound patterns. Am J Clin Pathol 52:258–269, 1969 and are reprinted here with the permission of the author, Rudiger Breitenecker, M.D., Baltimore, Maryland, the *American Journal of Clinical Pathology,* Dallas, Texas, and the Williams and Wilkins Company, Baltimore, Maryland.

a. **Long range wounds.**
   (1) When the charge has separated completely, each pellet striking the target causes an individual perforation. Wads frequently cause circular, nonpenetrating abrasions of the skin, but at this range do not enter the body.
   (2) When the charge has separated partially, it consists of a central aggregate of many pellets surrounded by a spread of individual pellets. This causes a complex wound pattern characterized by an irregular defect (usually 2 to 3 inches in diameter) with ragged margins ("rat hole") and surrounding satellite perforations. Wads may enter the body through the large defect or inflict nonpenetrating injuries.
b. **Intermediate range wounds.** In most instances, pellet dispersion begins at ranges of about 3 to 6 feet. Wounds at this range consist of defects with irregular margins, usually about 2 inches in diameter, with a few satellite perforations at the margins of the main defect. Characteristically wads enter the body through the large defect and no fouling is present.
c. **Close range wounds.** Pellets strike the target as a tightly knit mass and create a single defect, usually 1 to 1½ inches in diameter, with more or less smooth margins. The closer the range, the smaller the defect and the smoother the margins. Powder residue (fouling and stippling) is deposited on the target (see Chapter XXII, handgun injuries) and wads carry into the body.[4]
d. **Contact wounds.** The appearance of contact wounds is determined by the area of the body which is wounded and the tight-

---

[4] Editors note: Rarely scorching of the skin surrounding the wounds is noted. This is due to the large quantity of very hot gas emitted from the muzzle.

ness of contact between the end of the barrel and the skin. When skin is well supported and close to bone (*e.g.*, head), contact wounds are extensively lacerated. In the case of the head, expanding gas (produced by the combustion of gunpowder) and the pellets frequently have an explosive effect resulting in subtotal decapitation. ("He blew off the top of his head.") Contact wounds of the torso are smoothly marginated defects containing abundant powder residue. If contact is loose or if clothing is interposed between the end of the barrel and the skin, the skin adjacent to the perforation exhibits fouling. Wads always enter the body; occasionally they exit (see below). Contact wounds of the torso also exhibit localized pink discoloration of skeletal muscle due to the uptake of carbon monoxide and possibly also the presence of nitrites.[5]

5. **Exit wounds.** Generally shotgun pellets do not exit from the body. Exceptions are:
   a. Contact wounds of the head and trunk.
   b. Tangentially oriented wounds (contact or distant) where some of the pellets have a very short track through the body.
   c. Wounding of a thin part of the body such as the neck or extremities.
   d. Wounds inflicted by large caliber buckshot or rifled slugs.

Examination of the Body

Preliminary steps.

1. Examination of clothing is extremely important. Care must be exercised to avoid cutting or mutilating a wound pattern on clothing.
2. Good photography, including a scale for comparison with test patterns, is mandatory.

Autopsy.

1. Accurate description of the wound:
   a. Locate the central part of the wound with respect to an anatomic landmark as well as vertical (inches above the heel or below the top of the head) and horizontal (inches to the right or left of the midline) coordinates.
   b. Describe the character and size of the central skin defect and presence or absence of fouling and stippling (see handgun injuries, Chapter XXII).
   c. Describe the number and distribution of satellite skin perforations inflicted by individual pellets and the presence or absence of wad injuries.

---

[5] Editors note: The discoloration of skeletal muscle due to the combination of carbon monoxide with hemoglobin and myoglobin may occur at ranges up to several inches.

d. Measure the total vertical and horizontal spread of the skin wound pattern when satellite perforations are present.
2. Recovery of pellets and wads:
   a. With shot or small buckshot it is impractical (nearly impossible) to recover all of the pellets. A representative number (about 25) will allow the firearms expert to determine the average size and/or weight of the pellets. Small pellets are not marked for identification.
   b. With large buckshot it may be practical to recover all pellets, as there may be as few as six; x-ray is helpful in locating the buckshot. These are large enough to individually mark.
   c. Recovery of wads is mandatory; they reveal the gauge of the shotgun and may also have a manufacturer's mark. *Felt disks absorb blood and may be difficult to distinguish from clots.* Wads are not marked for identification.[6]
3. Specimens to save:
   a. Blood for typing.
   b. Blood, urine, or other appropriate specimens for toxicologic studies that may be indicated. In adults who do not survive their injuries for more than 18 to 24 hours, an analysis of blood for alcoholic content may yield useful information.

Special Procedures
1. Clothing must be preserved for comparison of wound patterns and for detection of powder residue.
2. There may be indications to examine the decedent's hands for evidence that he fired a gun or struggled to gain control of the shotgun responsible for the fatal shooting.

Pitfalls and Pearls
1. Do not overlook injuries unrelated to the shotgun wound. Is there evidence to suggest that the decedent was in a fight prior to being shot?
2. Precise estimates of the range of fire require that the wound pattern on the skin or clothing be compared with a series of experimental test patterns made by firing the same shotgun with the same ammunition as that involved in the fatality. Test shots are fired at appropriate targets until there is reasonable approximation of the pattern found on the victim's clothing or body.
3. Passage of shotgun pellets through any target before they strike the body causes the pellets to spread. This pertains to any intermediate object, no matter how thin, such as a window pane, screen, or layers of clothing. Therefore, one cannot compare experimental test

---

[6] Editors note: Felt wads wet with blood or other body fluids may swell and be distorted. They are best measured after drying. Plastic wads do not distort when immersed in fluid.

patterns with a wound pattern on the skin to estimate range if the charge passed through an intermediate target before striking the victim.

4. Spread of the pellets as seen by x-ray examination cannot be used to compare with test patterns to estimate range of fire. X-ray appearances may be similar in close and distant wounds even though the skin patterns may vary remarkably one from the other.

References

1. Breitenecker, R: Shotgun wound patterns. Am J Clin Pathol, 52:285–269, 1969

2. Breitenecker, R, Senior, W: I. Shotgun patterns. An experimental study on the influence of intermediate targets. Forensic Sci 12:193–204, 1967

3. Guerin, PF: Shotgun wounds. Forensic Sci 5:294–318, 1960

Chapter XXIV
CUTTING AND STABBING WOUNDS

Charles J. Stahl, Captain, MC, USN [1]
Chief, Forensic Sciences Division
Armed Forces Institute of Pathology
Washington, D.C.

Introduction

Definitions

a. **Incised wound.** An incised wound, incision, slash or cut is an injury caused by a sharp-edged instrument. The length of the wound is usually greater than the depth. Incised wounds are produced by instruments such as sharp knives, razor blades, or shards of glass. These wounds may have either smooth or irregular margins. Neither marginal abrasion nor undermining of the wound are evident. As the result of the pressure and the sharp edge of the instrument, bridging of subcutaneous tissue between the margins of the wound is absent (Figure 1).

b. **Stab wound.** A stab wound is a penetration of the body by a sharp and/or pointed instrument such as an ice pick, needle, knife, sword, or pointed rod. The depth of the wound is usually greater than the length. Abrasion of the margins of the wound is usually absent, except when a wound is inflicted with great force. The depth of the wound may be greater than the length of the instrument which inflicted the injury, depending upon the site and the degree of force. If the instrument is broken, a fragment of the instrument may be found. If the weapon has a sharp single-edged blade, one angle of the wound may appear slightly rounded or torn when compared to the opposite acute angle of the wound. If the instrument is withdrawn after the stab, an incision of the skin may be seen adjacent to the acute angle of the wound.

c. **Chop wound.** A deep, gaping wound, frequently involving major blood vessels, nerves, muscles, and bone, resulting from

---

[1] Editors note: The opinions or assertations contained here are the private views of the author and are not to be construed as official or as reflecting the views of the Department of Defense or of the Department of the Navy.

151

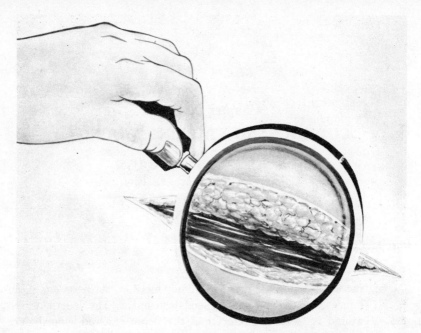

Figure 1: Diagram of an incised wound which has smooth, gaping margins. Note the absence of marginal abrasion, undermining of the wound, and bridging of tissues between the margins of the wound (AFIP Neg. No. 71–10832–2)

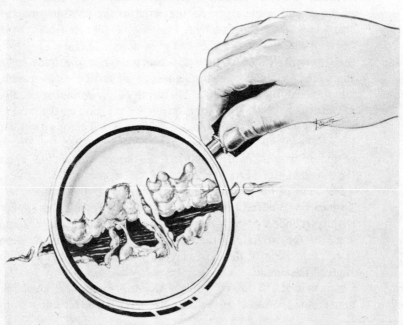

Figure 2: Diagram of a laceration which has irregular, undermined margins and shows bridging of skin and subcutaneous tissues between the margins of the wound (AFIP Neg. No. 71–10832–1)

an impact by a heavy, sharp-edged instrument such as an axe or machete.

d. **Laceration.** Lacerations are caused by impact with blunt objects, resulting in crushing, stretching and tearing. The wounds are frequently undermined and abraded. The margins of lacerations are irregular and bridging of tissue is observed between the margins (Figure 2).

The wound may contain foreign material from the impacting object. A laceration, or tear, is not an injury caused by a sharp-edged instrument, but this term is often used erroneously by pathologists to describe incised wounds.

2. **Classification of cutting and stabbing wounds.**
   a. **Therapeutic, or operative wounds.**
      (1) Surgical incision
      (2) Needle puncture
      (3) Incised (stab) wound for drainage
   b. **Accidental wounds.**
      (1) Fall upon a sharp-edged object
      (2) Impact by sharp objects such as fragments of glass
      (3) Unintentional cut or stab by sharp-edged and/or pointed instrument such as a tool, household utensil, knife, or razor blade.
   c. **Suicidal wounds.**
      (1) Superficial, multiple, parallel, and superimposed incisions of varying depth, known as hesitation wounds and often found on the forearms, neck, and legs.
      (2) Multiple sites of the body are frequently selected, and there may be scars of the neck and wrists, evidence of prior attempts at suicide.
      (3) In right-handed persons, the most severe wounds are often found on the left side of the body. Wounds of the neck are usually located above the thyroid cartilage and they are often deep, irregular, and obliquely oriented. The incision is deeper at the beginning of the cut and shallower at the end of the stroke.
      (4) Suicidal stab wounds are uncommon. Either the anterior surface of the chest or the abdomen are the usual sites. The depth of wounds must be determined because tentative or trial stab wounds are often superficial. If clothing is cut or if there are multiple, penetrating stab wounds in inaccessible sites, homicide should be suspected.
      (5) Persons who commit suicide may use more than one method to accomplish the act. If incised and/or stab wounds are superficial, consider the possibility of death resulting from a missile wound, drug, poison, etc.

153

d. **Homicidal wounds.**
  (1) Usually multiple, gaping wounds of the body, particularly the face, neck, chest, extremities, or back. Wounds of the face and neck are often deep. Hesitation wounds are not present.
  (2) As the result of attempts by the victim to protect himself, cuts of the posterior aspect of the forearms and the palmar surfaces of the fingers and hand, known as defense wounds, may be found.
  (3) Multiple, severe wounds resulting from mutilation of the body, particularly the breasts and genitalia, are consistent with sex-related murder. In men, similar wounds have resulted from homosexual rage.
e. **Postmortem wounds.**
  (1) Intentional mutilation
    (a) Sex crimes
    (b) Sadistic murder
    (c) Attempted concealment of body by dismemberment
    (d) Patterned, or symbolic wounds following torture or assassination
  (2) Unintentional mutilation
    Propellers of motor boats after drowning

3. **Complication and/or causes of death.**
  a. Hemorrhage
    (1) External
    (2) Internal
    (3) Intratracheal with asphyxia
  b. Air embolism
  c. Infection
  d. Hemopneumothorax

Preliminary Steps
1. **On-the-scene investigation.**
  a. Record the date, time, location, and environmental conditions.
  b. Obtain photographs to show the relationship of the body to the scene of death.
  c. Determine the presence or absence of the instrument used to inflict the injuries.
  d. Determine the presence or absence of letters or notes indicative of suicide.
  e. Describe the condition and state of preservation of the remains, as well as the position and condition of clothing.
  f. Review the investigative information provided by the law enforcement agency.
  g. Observe, describe, record, and photograph stains of blood and

154

other body fluids in relationship to the remains and the scene of death.

   h. Participate in the evaluation of physical evidence, including collection of weapons, containers with drugs, and biological stains.

   i. Establish and maintain chain of custody for physical evidence.

   j. Prepare diagrams or drawings of the scene.

2. **Establish objectives.**

   a. Identification of the victim

   b. Cause of death

   c. Manner of death

   d. Estimation of time of death

   e. Estimation of duration of survival after injury, including the possibility of volitional acts by the victim.

   f. Classification of each wound, as well as the relationship of the wound to defects in the clothing and the type of instrument required to cause the wound.

   g. Determination of the direction and depth and estimation of the force required to cause each wound.

   h. Distinction between antemortem and postmortem injuries.

   i. Recognition of artifacts.

   j. Collection of physical evidence resulting from interchange of hair, blood, fibers, and body fluids between the assailant and the victim. Establish and maintain the chain of custody for this evidence.

Autopsy

1. **Preliminary procedures.**

   a. Obtain photographs prior to and during the autopsy, including close-up photographs of selected wounds and defects in clothing.

   b. Examine, carefully remove, and describe the clothing. Do not cut or tear the clothing. Correlate defects in clothing with wounds. If clothing is wet or bloodstained, carefully hang it to air dry. Retain as evidence for subsequent examination by crime laboratory.

   c. Identify the victim.

   d. Obtain samples of hair from the head and pubic area, as well as samples of blood and fingernail scrapings or clippings for subsequent examinations.

   e. Examine genitalia, anal area, and oral cavity for evidence of rape or other sexual assaults. Collect and retain appropriate specimens as evidence for subsequent examinations.

   f. Determine presence or absence of foreign material such as fragments of glass or metal. Do not insert a probe into wounds. Obtain x-rays of wounded body areas.

g. Review hospital records and operative reports to determine the location of therapeutic needle marks, surgical incisions, and operative procedures.

h. Review a textbook of anatomy to relate the location of the wounds to Langer's lines of cleavage. Elastic fibers in the skin provide tension and smoothness. Incised wounds, parallel to the lines of cleavage, do not tend to gape. When elastic fibers are severed by an incision perpendicular to the lines of cleavage, gaping is evident (Figure 3).

2. **Examine and describe the external injuries.**

   a. Correlate the injuries with defects in the clothing.

   b. Determine the anatomic site, width, length, depth, shape, and direction of each wound. Obtain x-rays and photographs as necessary. Do not probe or insert the weapon into the wound.

   c. Determine the height of the victim and prepare diagrams to show the anatomic relationships of the wounds to the distance from the feet and/or the top of the head.

   d. Determine the type of each wound. It may be useful to employ a hand lens to distinguish cutting and stabbing wounds from lacerations. Examine for distinctive patterns of injury which may be related to suspected weapons.

   e. Determine if defensive wounds or hesitation wounds are present.

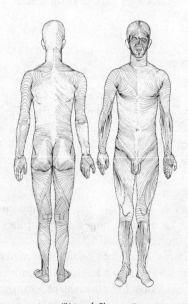

"Lines of Cleavage"

Figure 3: Diagram of Langer's lines. (AFIP Neg. No. 69–2899–1)

f. Examine concealed sites such as the eyes, oral cavity, scalp, genital region, and base of the neck.
g. Examine, describe, record, and photograph other related external injuries such as gunshot wounds or blunt force injuries.

3. **Examine and describe the internal injuries.**
a. Carefully proceed with the internal examination to determine whether or not the cutting or stabbing wounds could have resulted in air embolism. Also, determine if pneumothorax is present.
b. Correlate the direction, track, and site of internal injuries with the external wounds and defects in the clothing. Obtain x-rays and photographs, as necessary.
c. Determine the length of the track for each penetrating wound, the relationship of the wound to bony structures, and the type of weapon or instrument consistent with the wound.
d. Determine if multiple thrusts of the instrument were made through a single stab wound.
e. Determine the location and amount of hemorrhage into body cavities. Measure the amount of blood.
f. Recognition artifacts.
g. Determine the presence or absence of other types of injuries or significant pre-existing diseases, as well as the effects of prior diagnostic, therapeutic, or operative procedures.
h. Determine which wounds resulted in death of the victim.
i. Collect and preserve by freezing, samples of blood, bile, urine, gastric contents, and organs for subsequent toxicologic examinations.
j. After all external, internal, photographic, and radiographic studies have been completed, excise selected wounds for microscopic examination.

Special Procedures

1. **Microscopic examination.**
a. Confirmation and diagnosis of pre-existing natural diseases.
b. Estimation of age of injuries.
c. Detection of foreign material.
d. Evaluation of the complications of cutting and stabbing wounds such as extent of hemorrhage, infection, infarction, and thrombosis.
e. Distinguish between antemortem and postmortem injuries.
f. Evaluation of other traumatic injuries.

2. **Diagrams.**
a. Anatomic diagrams or drawings of wounds.
b. Tracings of wounds *in situ* on plastic film.

157

288-953 O - 79 - 11

3. **Casts of wounds.**
   a. Use dental impression material to obtain cast.
   b. Use plaster of Paris to prepare a positive mold from the cast.
4. **Radiographic studies.**
   a. Soft x-ray.
   b. Instillation of radio-opaque media into track.
   c. X-ray diffraction studies of foreign materials.
5. **Toxicologic studies.**
6. **Criminalistic studies.**
   a. Determination of blood group and blood type of victim.
   b. Evaluation of stains of blood and body fluids.
   c. Comparative examination of hair and fibers.
   d. Fingerprints.
   e. Evaluation of fingernail scrapings and clippings.
   f. Examination of suspected weapons and of clothing.

Pitfalls—Do's and Don'ts

1. Distinguish between incised wounds and lacerations.
2. Recognize therapeutic or operative wounds.
3. Distinguish between antemortem and postmortem injuries.
4. Recognize defense wounds and hesitation wounds.
5. Examine clothing of the victim and correlate the defects with the wounds.
6. Obtain photographs and x-rays.
7. Examine, describe, record, and photograph wounds to determine anatomic location, size, shape, and type, as well as to determine direction and to estimate force required to cause the wound.
8. Collect and retain hair, stains, fingernail scrapings and clippings, and other physical evidence, as well as appropriate specimens for toxicologic and serologic examinations.
9. Consider the possibility of air embolism.
10. Establish and maintain chain of custody for physical evidence.
11. Do not probe the wounds prior to careful external and/or internal examination.
12. Do not insert the weapon into the wound.
13. Do not provide a dogmatic opinion concerning the length of the blade and type of weapon used to inflict the wound.
14. Do not place specimens for toxicologic and serologic studies in formalin solution.
15. Do not forward wet, bloodstained clothing to the crime laboratory.
16. Do not exclude the possibility of suicide when multiple cutting and stabbing wounds are found in regions of the neck, trunk and extremities accessible to the victim.
17. Do not fail to recognize postmortem artifacts.

158

18. Do not confuse more than one adjacent cut in clothing or skin as two stab wounds, for in a single thrust the blade may pass through folds of clothing or skin.
19. Do not exclude the possibility of other causes for death such as drugs, poisons, drowning, or natural disease.
20. Do not fail to consider accidental injuries, resulting in cuts or stabs which may occur at work or in the home.

Chapter XXV

BLUNT TRAUMA—GENERAL

Jerry T. Francisco, M.D.
Chief Medical Examiner
State of Tennessee
Memphis, Tennessee

Introduction

Incidence. The autopsy in a medicolegal case has several special parameters. None are more crucial and more difficult than the evaluations of blunt trauma. These include answering several questions:

1. How did the trauma occur?
2. Did it occur before or after death, and if before, how long before?
3. What is its significance in relation to the cause of death?
4. What object or objects could have produced it?
5. What was the vector of force?
6. How much force was required to produce it?

In order to answer these questions the medicolegal autopsy must be very detailed. There must be: (1) a precise description of the wounds; (2) photographs of the wounds (including a scale of size); and (3) diagrams, prepared to scale, which identify the anatomical locations and sizes of the wounds present.

Mechanisms of Production

A knowledge of wound production is necessary to interpret wounds caused by blunt trauma and to answer the above questions.

Principles involved. Blunt or mechanical injury is produced when sufficient energy is absorbed so that there is permanent alteration of some part of the body's anatomic integrity. The result is a wound.

Injuries may be wounds, but not necessarily. This chapter will be confined to wounds.

2. **Energy available.** The available energy is determined by the products of mass and its velocity. This is expressed by the formula $E = MV^2$. Gravity acts to diminish the effects of lateral velocity and thus the complete formula is: $E = M \dfrac{v^2}{2g}$, where $g =$ the acceleration of gravity.

160

3. **Energy transferred.** Regardless of the amount of available energy, unless it is transferred to the body no wound will result. The following factors act to determine the speed with which energy is transferred.

a. **Area of application.** The area over the body to which the energy is transferred is of significance. Thus, energy applied to a small area is more likely to produce a wound than an equal amount applied to a larger area.

b. **Time of transfer.** The body has a certain capacity to absorb energy. Therefore, a rapid transfer of energy is more likely to produce a wound than a slow transfer.

4. **Energy absorbed.** It is not the total amount of energy absorbed by the body as a whole that is significant in production of a wound, but the amount localized in one area that is significant. The area of application is thus modified by several special features of the tissues and physical principles.

a. **Lever action.** Certain parts of the body are constructed to make use of lever action. These portions are thus susceptible to a concentration of total energy transferred (*i.e.,* the elbow in a blow to the palm of the outstretched arm.)

b. **Plasticity and elasticity.** Certain parts of the body can be bent, twisted, or compressed and not wounded. The elastic tissue of the dermis is an example. A force may injure underlying organs but not damage the skin. Injury to a lung of a child without fracture of ribs is another example.

c. **Inertia.** If a part of the body is relatively fixed, its inertia will be high. Because the anatomic part will resist movement all energy absorbed will be of wounding force. Two examples of fixation of organs are the ligament of Treitz on the small intestine and the aorta distal to the origin of the great vessels.

d. **Hydrostatic pressure.** In fluid filled organs such as blood vessels, a type of lever action occurs so that energy may be magnified with a resulting contusion and on occasion, rupture.

In summation the formula can be presented as: $W = E \times \frac{1}{T} \times \frac{1}{A} \times k$, with W = wound, E = energy available, T = period of energy transfer, A = area of application, and K = modifying factors for area and period of energy transfer.

Examination of Skin

A skin wound must be very carefully examined and described. Photographs and accurate diagrams are important in documenting the injury and should be included as a part of the written record.

1. **Type of object.** The object causing the wound may leave an imprint which may be helpful in identifying it (*i.e.,* the grill of a motor vehicle may produce a patterned abrasion on the skin).

161

2. **Direction of force.** The direction from which the force is applied may be determined by a careful examination of the skin. The fact that trauma has been sustained is a very obvious reason for a detailed examination of the skin. It is often as significant to document this as to determine the cause of death. This is one of the most overlooked phases of a medicolegal autopsy.

Types of Wounds

It is most important to define and identify precisely the type of wound present. Physicians have a tendency to use words interchangeably. Obviously this should be avoided in medicolegal practice.

1. **Abrasion.** This is a wound produced by friction or scraping. It may be superficial or deep. It most frequently involves skin but occasionally may involve other organs. This type of wound is most helpful in determining the direction of force because the surface layers will be "piled up" on the side opposite the direction of force.

The dermis in a postmortem abrasion will be brown in color, whereas a premortem abrasion will have a red color. (Vital vascular reaction causes the red color to show.)

2. **Contusion.** The contusion is a rupturing of blood vessels of an organ due to the hydrostatic forces effect from trauma. A hematoma occurs when the bleeding from these vessels is rapid.

3. **Laceration.** This is tearing of tissue resulting from excessive stretching. This tearing may leave strands of tissue in the depths of the wound which are unbroken and "bridge" the edges of the wound. The laceration is usually perpendicular to the vector of force producing it. On the head the laceration will be stellate if the force is perpendicular to the plane that produces a tangent with the skull. It must be distinguished from an incision.

4. **Incision.** A cut. Avoid the bad habit of using laceration and incision interchangeably.

5. **Fracture.** A fracture is functionally a laceration of a bone. Many attorneys are under the impression that radiographic examination is a better way of demonstrating fractures than by direct observation.[1] The type and location of a fracture can be of use in indicating the direction of force or may suggest the wounding object. "Bumper fractures" are often bilateral fractures of the tibia and fibula in the middle one-third of their shafts resulting from an automobile bumper striking the lower extremity.

6. **Special mechanism of wounds.**

a. **Cerebral contusions.** It is a well established fact that contusions to the cerebral tissue have patterns which may be very helpful. If the

---

[1] Editors note: Many fractures, particularly of bones of the skull, are not well demonstrated by x-ray. Indeed, a sizeable percentage of skull fractures cannot be seen in the usual methods of x-ray examination of the skull.

162

moving head strikes a fixed object (*i.e.,* falls) than the cerebral contusions resulting from this trauma will be more severe on the point of the brain that is contralateral from the skin damage (contrecoup). If the fixed head is struck by a moving object (*i.e.,* blow) then the opposite is true; the cerebral damage will be more severe on the side with the skin damage (coup). The mechanisms are in dispute but the observation is clear.[2]

Foreign Particles

1. In any wound a search should be made for any foreign materials. This may help to identify the object which caused the wound. Glass from an automobile head lamp may be embedded in the wounds of the pedestrian. A knife tip may be broken off in a stab wound. Wire fragments may be embedded in the skin when a gun is fired through screen wire.

2. The examination of these wounds should be performed with a hand lens or a dissecting microscopue. In certain cases this may be the most important part of the autopsy.

Do's and Don'ts

1. Do carefully examine the skin.
2. Do diagram, photograph, and describe all skin wounds no matter how minor.
3. Do look for and retain foreign debris found in wounds.
4. Do not confuse a postmortem wound with an antemortem wound.
5. Do not use words such as laceration and incision interchangeably.

References

1. Moritz, AR, Adelson, L: Physical agents in causation of injury and disease, Pathology of Trauma. Sixth edition. Edited by WAD Anderson. The CV Mosby Company, St. Louis, 1971, pp 145–173
2. Petty, CS: Soft tissue injuries: an overview. J Trauma, 10:201–219, 1970
3. Spitz, WU: Blunt force injury, Medicolegal Investigation of Death. Edited by WU Spitz, RS Fisher. Charles C Thomas, Springfield, 1973, pp 122–150

---

[2] Editors note: Beware the head injury produced by a "compound" type of injury: both the "moving head" and "fixed head" types of cerebral contusions are present. Such injuries are difficult if not impossible to interpret.

Chapter XXVI
BLUNT TRAUMA: SPECIFIC INJURIES

Michael M. Baden, M.D.
Deputy Chief Medical Examiner
New York, New York
and
Charles S. Petty, M.D.
Chief Medical Examiner of Dallas County
Director, Southwestern Institute of Forensic Sciences
Dallas, Texas

Introduction

1. Blunt trauma can be generalized or localized.
    a. Generalized: involving multiple areas of the body, *e.g.,* fall from heights (building, bridge); vehicular accidents (see Chapter XXXI).
    b. Localized: involving one or two areas of the body, *e.g.,* fall down stairs or while walking; blow with a weapon; crush injuries, as by an elevator.
2. Sometimes specific imprints of an impacting object may be identified on the skin, *e.g.,* pipe threads, automobile radiator grill.
3. Fatal injuries resulting from blunt trauma usually are nonspecific: diffuse ecchymoses, fractures of bones, and lacerations of viscera.

Preliminary Steps

1. Complete information regarding the circumstances of death is critical. It may be difficult to determine at autopsy whether someone has fallen from a height or has been struck by an automobile.
2. Clothing should be examined for trace evidence, tire marks, patterned abrasions and object imprints.
3. In falls from heights, inquiry should be made regarding any history of depression or the presence of a suicide note. Examination of the scene where the body was found, the place from which the deceased fell, and the residence of the deceased may contribute to ascertaining the manner of death (suicide, accident, homicide).

Autopsy

1. Generalized blunt force injuries: contusions, abrasions, and lacera-

tions of the skin are described in Chapter XXV. No external evidence of trauma may be evident despite extensive internal injuries. This sometimes obtains in instances of falls from great heights. Internal injuries can include multiple fractures of the skull, ribs, long bones, pelvis, and spine. Contusions of the brain and lacerations of the internal viscera, most frequently the lungs, liver, spleen, mesentery, and heart may be seen at autopsy. Internal herniation of abdominal viscera through a torn diaphragm may also occur. Fractured ribs may lacerate the lungs; pelvic fractures may be associated with laceration of the urinary bladder and/or urethra; fractures of the skull with even momentary depression of the bony fragments may lacerate the brain. Thus injury to one tissue or organ may result in a "secondary" injury to another.

2. Localized blunt force injuries: isolated injuries of the liver, spleen or other viscera from localized trauma to the abdomen can cause death by internal hemorrhage. Most localized blunt force injuries that prove fatal involve the head and cause intracranial bleeding including epidural, subdural, subarachnoid, and intracerebral hemorrhages.
   a. Head injuries.
      (1) Subdural hemorrhages are almost always produced by trauma. Those that are fatal are frequently associated with contusions or lacerations of the brain and fractures of the skull. A fatal head injury sustained in a fall often involves force applied to the occipital area. The moving head strikes the hard and unyielding surface. The scalp and skull are damaged most frequently in the occipital area; the frontal and temporal poles of the brain are contused. (See contrecoup injury in Chapter XXV.) These findings alone will not resolve whether the deceased fell accidentally or was pushed during an assault. Knowledge of the circumstances is necessary to determine the manner of death. A direct blow to the stationary head with a weapon can produce a skull fracture at the impact site and ipsilateral cerebral injury and hemorrhage (coup injury). A skull fracture is seldom present when a traumatic subdural hemorrhage results from the tearing of a communicating or meningeal vessel without underlying cerebral parenchymal injury. Occasionally a large spontaneous subarachnoid hemorrhage can rupture through the leptomeninges into the subdural space and produce a nontraumatic subdural clot. This must always be considered by the prosector.
      (2) Epidural hemorrhage is always traumatic and usually associated with a fracture of a bone that lacerates a branch of the middle meningeal artery.
      (3) Subarachnoid hemorrhage not associated with cerebral in-

jury is almost always spontaneous, often due to rupture of a saccular (berry) aneurysm of an artery of the Circle of Willis, or a branch thereof, or another artery at the base of the brain.

(4) Intracerebral hemorrhage can be spontaneous (hypertensive, arteriosclerotic) or traumatic. The latter is usually consequent to direct laceration of the brain associated with a skull fracture, to distortion of the brain by outside force, or to internal compression against dural margins (such as, the tentorium cerebelli with resultant lacerations of the cerebral peduncles or pons).

b. Neck injuries of the type incurred in a fall down stairs can include fractures and dislocations of the cervical vertebrae and compression or laceration of the spinal cord. A blow to the lateral aspect of the upper neck can cause a traumatic subarachnoid hemorrhage extending to the base of the brain due to fracture of a proximal cervical vertebra and associated laceration of the vertebral artery. In such an injury, the vertebral artery is lacerated in its intraforaminal portion.

c. Compression of the chest of a severe and prolonged type will result in prominent cyanosis and petechiae in the skin above the level of compression and death by traumatic asphyxia. If the injured person survives such injury, lower nephron nephrosis may develop and cause death.

3. Delayed sequellae of blunt trauma.
   a. Pulmonary thromboemboli, marrow or fat emboli may result from blunt force injuries. Fractures and surgical manipulation of long bones may cause the latter. Fat emboli can cause petechiae in the skin and conjunctivae and fat can be identified in the clinical laboratory in urine and cerebrospinal fluid. Sections of the lungs, brain or kidneys taken at autopsy, stained to demonstrate fat, may reveal fat emboli.
   b. Localized infection from penetrating injuries and pneumonia or pyelonephritis developing during bed rest are also expected sequellae of injury.
   c. Excessive callus formation of a healing vertebral fracture can cause encroachment upon the spinal cord and delayed compression of the spinal cord and paraplegia.
   d. Acute cerebral compression from subdural hemorrhage or cerebral edema can cause secondary cerebral infarctions, especially of the medial occipital lobe cortex due to compression of the posterior cerebral vessels against dural margins.
   e. As noted above, lower nephron nephrosis may result, particularly if there has been much crushing of the muscle and release of myoglobin into the blood stream.

166

f. Frequently overlooked is delayed rupture of viscera, *e.g.,* the spleen or aorta. Such viscera, injured at the time of the traumatic incident may well retain overall integrity until much later when rupture and fatal hemorrhage results. Intervals of days to several weeks between injury and rupture have been recorded many times.

Special Procedures

1. Determine the blood (vitreous humor, cerebrospinal fluid, or other body fluid) alcohol content. If there is a possibility of suicide or drug abuse, appropriate toxicologic investigation should be undertaken.
2. Occasionally analysis of a subdural hematoma or other sequestered blood clot for alcohol or carbon monoxide (carboxyhemoglobin) content may prove of value.
3. Photographs should be taken of significant injuries, especially external patterned injuries.
4. Diagrams indicating the location, nature and extent of injuries may be of value. These are especially useful to establish injury patterns.

Do's and Don'ts

1. Do not assume that little external evidence of trauma is necessarily associated with little internal trauma.
2. Do obtain a complete history and reports of police investigations. Autopsy alone often cannot reveal whether the blunt force injuries are the result of homicide, suicide, or accident.

Chapter XXVII
DRUG DEATHS BY INJECTION

Charles S. Hirsch, M.D.
Associate Pathologist and Deputy Coroner
Cuyahoga County Coroner's Office
Cleveland, Ohio

Introduction

Apparatus and preparation of drugs for injection. Illicit narcotics are purchased "on the street" as packets of powder containing the alkaloid (usually 4 to 8 percent) which has been diluted ("cut") by quinine, lactose, mannitol or some other adulterant.[1] The powder is prepared for injection by placing it in tap water in a suitable small receptacle such as a bottle cap or spoon ("cooker"). The bottom of the "cooker" is heated until the powder dissolves. The solution is then drawn into a standard or improvised syringe, often through a bit of cotton to filter out insoluble particles. Belts or elastic bands are employed as tourniquets to facilitate intravenous injection. Many addicts make "syringes" by fixing a hypodermic needle to a medicine dropper. The distal end of the dropper is often wound with a fragment of cloth or paper which acts as a flange for improving the snugness of fit with the needle hub.

As most addicts are unfamiliar with or inattentive to sterile technics, their apparatus is usually grossly contaminated. Communal use of equipment is common.

The drug solutions often contain insoluble, crystalline particles of microscopic size. The amount of crystalline debris is greatly increased in instances when the addict injects solutions prepared from tablets or capsules intended for oral consumption (*e.g.,* Ritalin or "west coast").

Intravenous injection sites ("mainlining"). The most common primary injection site is the antecubital region. As veins become unusable ("burned out"), addicts inject veins on the dorsum of the hand, foot, or almost any other conceivable location.

Characteristic lesions ("tracers") are hyperpigmented linear scars overlying sclerotic subcutaneous veins. Punctate areas of black discoloration ("soot tattooing") are caused by deposition of carbonaceous material

---

[1] Editors note: Frequently (in some parts of the country) cut with methapyrilene.

along the track of the needle. Such debris adheres to the needle when it is flamed in a makeshift attempt at sterilization.

Addicts may conceal tracers with tattoos; and they sometimes try to obliterate them by abrading, burning, or by otherwise scarifying the area.

Subcutaneous or intramuscular injection sites ("skin popping"). Skin popping (injection without intent to enter a vein) allegedly is used by a greater number of female than male addicts. Neophytes may begin by skin popping, and long-term mainliners may be forced to return to skin popping when their accessible subcutaneous veins are no longer usable. Customary target areas are the upper arms and thighs; however, any fold of skin or mucous membrane may be used (including nasal and oral mucous membranes).

Recent injection sites generally are characterized by zones of inflammation surrounding or adjacent to a needle puncture site. The inflammatory foci may resolve leaving no trace, or may form abscesses or ulcerations. Healing by fibrosis may produce hyperpigmented macules or retracted, circumscribed scars which resemble those from smallpox vaccinations.

Preliminary Steps

If drug packets or injection paraphernalia are recovered at the scene of death or from the decedent's clothing, retain them for chemical studies.

Autopsy

The addict with characteristic skin lesions is recognized easily. *However, cutaneous stigmata of addiction or narcotic abuse may be entirely absent.*

Method of examination for intravenous injections. A suitable method of examination is to make a single longitudinal incision of the flexor surface of each arm from mid-bicep to distal forearm. Using sharp or blunt dissection and staying close to the deep surface of the skin, the incised margins are reflected widely to expose subcutaneous tissue and veins. Artifactual hemorrhage is reduced if the veins are decompressed by waiting to dissect the arms until the thoracic viscera have been removed.

Examination of the arms by this technic in suspected narcotic deaths offers a number of advantages: (1) recent and resolving subcutaneous hemorrhages, and their relationship to veins, are documented unequivocally; (2) long segments of the veins favored by most addicts are exposed; and (3) perivenous inflammatory changes and pathologic changes in veins can be evaluated adequately. The dissection produces no significant cosmetic defect insofar as display of the body during the funeral services is concerned.

Specimens to be saved for chemical analysis.

1. Blood. (Narcotics or adulterants may not be easily demonstrable in blood).[2]
2. All available urine.   '
3. All available bile.
4. Liver, kidney, lung, and brain.
5. If dissection of the arms discloses a fresh subcutaneous extravasation of blood adjacent to a vein, excise the entire area and save the tissue in a chemically clean container. The toxicologist may be able to identify an adulterant (quinine, etc.) or even the narcotic itself in this specimen because of drug extravasation at the time of the injection.[3]

Findings at autopsy

1. Skin:
   a. Recent and resolving perivenous hemorrhage.
   b. Phlebitis, phlebosclerosis, and thrombosis.
   c. Suppurative or aseptic subcutaneous inflammation with or without foreign body granulomata (examine under polarized light).
   d. Black debris in the dermis which characteristically does not elicit an inflammatory reaction ("soot tattooing").
   e. Subcutaneous fibrosis with tiny areas of residual chronic inflammation or foreign body granulomata (examine under polarized light).
2. Lung: marked edema with or without hemorrhage and frequently with acute bronchopneumonia (examine under polarized light).
3. Liver: nonspecific, widespread lymphocytic infiltrates in portal areas.
4. Lymph nodes: characteristically enlarged at the porta hepatis and adjacent to the common bile duct. Microscopically nonspecific hyperplasia is seen.
5. Other life-threatening complications:
   a. Viral hepatitis
   b. Bacterial endocarditis (right or left side of the heart)
   c. Subcutaneous or lung abscess with septicemia
   d. Pulmonary angiothrombosis with foreign body granulomata and cor pulmonale
   e. Malaria
   f. Tetanus
   g. Syphilis
   h. Crush syndrome with myoglobinuric nephrosis

---

[2] Editors note: A well-equipped toxicology laboratory utilizing spectrophotometry and radioimmunoassay should be able to detect and quantitate very small amounts of morphine in blood samples.

[3] Editors note: A decision must first be made as to the relative value of preserving the tissue for toxicologic analysis, or using it for microscopic examination, or dividing it so as to accomplish both objectives.

Pitfalls and Pearls

Narcotic addicts are not immune to sudden and unexpected death caused by disease entirely unrelated to their addiction. A diagnosis of death due to narcotism rests upon a considered evaluation of information derived from all available sources, including thorough study of circumstances surrounding death, complete gross and microscopic anatomic examination, and indicated chemical studies.

Interpretation of the chronology of subcutaneous hemorrhages must be approached cautiously. Unless dry blood is present on the skin surface, there is no assurance that a fresh subcutaneous hemorrhage immediately preceded death.

Addicts frequently are "dumped" in public places after they die suddenly and unexpectedly on private premises ("shooting galleries"). The presence of milk in the victim's airway or rectum indicates that his companions attempted to resuscitate him.

Young persons who are killed while carrying out robberies or burglaries and prostitutes who die of violence should be autopsied, keeping narcotic addiction in mind.

References

1. Castleman, B, McNeely, BU: Case records of the Massachusetts General Hospital (Case 26–1971). N Eng J Med, 285:40–48, 1971

2. Gross, EM: Symposium: Pathology of narcotics and addictive drugs. Human Pathol, 3:11–112, 1972

3. Louria, DB, Hensle, T, Rose, J: The major medical complications of heroin addiction. Ann Intern Med, 67:1–22, 1967

4. Siegle, H, Bloustein, P: Continuing studies in the diagnosis and pathology of death from intravenous narcotism. J Forensic Sci, 15:179–184, 1970

5. Siegel, H, Helpern, M, Ehrenreich, T: The diagnosis of death from intravenous narcotism. J Forensic Sci, 11:1–16, 1966

Chapter XXVIII

DEATHS BY INHALATION OR INGESTION OF DRUGS AND OTHER POISONS

Allan B. McNie, M.D.
Pathologist, Institute of Forensic Sciences
Oakland, California

Introduction, Concepts, and Principles

1. Drug deaths are encountered frequently in all parts of the country
   a. The incidence is about 150 deaths per 1,000,000 population per year (Alameda County, California)
   b. It s a contributing factor in many additional deaths (*e.g.,* auto accidents, homicides, and suicides)
   c. Regional variation is quite apparent, and changes from time to time. The following may serve as examples:
      (1) Cyanide in the New England jewelry industry
      (2) Narcotics in seaport cities
      (3) Seconal on the West Coast
      (4) Thallium on the East Coast
      (5) Strychnine on the West Coast
      (6) Quinine on the East Coast from heroin
2. Number of drugs and drug-usage is increasing
   a. Any drug, prescription or otherwise, can cause death in certain circumstances
   b. Analytic methods may lag behind usage
   c. Drugs may inhibit or accelerate metabolism of other drugs
   d. Concept of poly-pharmacy, small amounts of many drugs, can be lethal
   e. Old drugs may be used in new ways
   f. Drug formulation may predispose to abuse
   g. Reported cases of drug deaths may lag behind the actual number of deaths
   h. Illicit manufacturing is a problem
   i. Drug deaths may occur in epidemics (*e.g.,* deaths from heroin or from methyl alcohol)
3. Finding of cases is proportional to the amount of interest and quality of the toxicologic examination.
   a. Drug screen should be done in all victims of homicide

172

b. Analysis for sedatives should be performed in all instances of asphyxia from a plastic bag and in bathtub drownings

c. Drug usage is often associated with fatal automobile crashes involving teenagers

d. Review of analytic schema periodically is necessary

4. Investigation of drug deaths involves *teamwork.*

    a. **Investigator.** Should observe and investigate the following:

        (1) drugs available

        (2) circumstances

        (3) appearance and position of body

        (4) all prescription items found must be checked with pharmacist

    b. **Pathologist.** Must do a complete autopsy in every case regardless of history. This will enable him to:

        (1) collect proper specimens for toxicologic examination

        (2) recognize drug cases

        (3) lend direction to the toxicologist (*e.g.,* hints from gross autopsy findings; type of drug screen desired)

    c. **Toxicologist.**

        (1) should review case with pathologist

        (2) should proceed with analyses in orderly manner

        (3) should always first look for drugs most frequently encountered

        (4) should discuss all interpretation of toxicologic findings with pathologist

5. Individual response to drugs varies greatly

    a. Tolerance

    b. Tenfold variation in some drugs (*i.e.,* barbiturates)

    c. Specific analytical methods are needed (the type of barbiturate must be known in order to interpret level)

    d. Presence of certain diseases may influence level of drug found at death

    e. Knowledge of the circumstances surrounding death is helpful in the interpretation of levels of drug

    f. Long-term drug therapy (or even misuse) may cause high non-lethal drug level

6. Deaths may occur a long time after ingestion of drugs; long after the drugs have disappeared from the system and from apparent unrelated causes

    a. Bronchopneumonia

    b. Therapeutic complications

        (1) air embolism

        (2) hemorrhage from tracheostomy

    c. Hepatitis

    d. Fungal or bacterial endocarditis

288-953 O - 79 - 12

e. Hematologic problems
f. Encephalomalacia
7. Levels of drug, less than lethal, may trigger other mechanisms of death
   a. Positional aspyhxia
   b. Intravascular sickling in certain hemoglobinopathies
   c. Postictal respiratory failure

Preliminary Steps
1. Competent death scene investigation
   a. History of despondency or previous attempts at suicide
   b. Any and all prescription medicines, not just those next to the body
   c. Check for glasses, bottles, pills, etc.
   d. Look for suicide notes not only in open view but also in waste baskets, trash cans, etc. Family may try to destroy note or other evidence
   e. Note the appearance and position of the body
   f. Determine when deceased was last seen alive
2. Deaths occurring after hospitalization
   a. Check clinical course for compatibility with drug overdose
   b. Check emergency room to see if gastric lavage was done and if the specimen is still available for analysis
   c. Check the clinical laboratory to see if any blood samples from admission may still be held in the refrigerator
   d. Check the record for reports of drug levels
3. Suspected deaths from drugs
   a. All cases where the history suggests involvement of drugs
   b. Deaths in teenagers and young adults without a history of pre-existing serious diseases
   c. Deaths in people with certain high-risk characteristics
      (1) *Physical stigmata* (*e.g.*, wrist scars, tracks and skin-pops, tattoos, etc.)
      (2) *Social groups with high drug use* (*e.g.*, motorcycle gangs; "hippies"; cults; etc.)
4. Have proper containers for specimens and maintain chain of custody
   a. Do not cross-contaminate specimens
   b. Properly identify with waterproof labels
   c. Properly seal to preserve chain of possession
   d. Do not re-use containers; use new plastic bags, plastic screw cap bottles, vacutainer tubes, etc.
   e. Always measure stomach contents. Take all or aliquot
   f. Consider need for "Special Specimens" (See Special Procedures)
   g. Provide for orderly accession to the laboratory and maintain chain of possession

Autopsy
1. External examination
   a. Look for tracks or evidence of skin popping; indication of an individual who abuses all types of drugs, not just narcotics
   b. Perforation of nasal septum
   c. Old scars from previous suicide attempts
   d. Burns about the mouth and lips from corrosives
   e. Postmortem lividity will be cherry red in carbon monoxide and cynaide poisoning and is hard to see in darkly pigmented people; mimicked by arterialized blood in exposure
   f. Blisters on extremities from barbiturates, sedatives, carbon monoxide, etc.
2. Characteristic odors
   a. May be strongest in stomach
   b. Compress chest sharply and inhale near nostril
      (1) alcohol
      (2) oil of wintergreen
      (3) cyanide—with inheritable trait some cannot smell [1]
      (4) paraldehyde
      (5) ethchlorvynol
      (6) petroleum products
      (7) nicotine
3. Internal examination: "Warning Signals"
   a. **Lungs congestion and edema.** Usually of significant amount. If heart disease and intracranial lesions are excluded, drugs are probable cause
   b. **Chemical gastritis.** Most commonly seen with barbiturates— usually in fundic or prepyloric area
   c. **Brain changes.**
      (1) Acute, may be swelling or pressure cone
      (2) Late, may be laminar necrosis or symmetrical necrosis of basal ganglia
   d. **Laryngeal edema.** Frequently seen in deaths from alcohol and barbiturate
   e. **Bladder.** Frequently very distended and often the only clue to death from drugs
   f. **Intravascular sickling.** May be triggered by drug ingestion
4. Collection of proper specimens should be routine in all cases
   a. Blood
      (1) collect specimen from heart in a clean container
      (2) collect at least 4 ounces
      (3) do not mix with pericardial fluid
      (4) do not collect from the chest cavity

---

[1] Editors note: Apparently 20 to 25 percent of all people cannot detect and recognize cyanide by smell.

   (5) blood from extremities is good source and may be obtained by elevating and aspirating from cut vessels even after evisceration

  b. Urine

   (1) collect 4 ounces (or whatever is available) in a clean container (1 to 2 cc. is enough for certain screening tests)

  c. Liver

   (1) take 500 grams

   (2) put in a separate plastic bag

   (3) store frozen if not needed immediately

  d. Stomach contents

   (1) take all if only small amount is present; if there is a large amount, take an aliquot

   (2) always measure contents

   (3) look for intact tablets or capsules which may suggest type of drug ingested

5. Before terminating autopsy

  a. Inject carotid arteries with water to determine patency

  b. Inspect uvula, pituitary, and middle ears

  c. When there are no specific findings consider the following:

   (1) seizure disorder

   (2) delirium tremens

   (3) electrolyte imbalance

   (4) positional asphyxia

   (5) intravascular sickling

Special Procedures—In addition to routine examinations

1. Narcotic cases

  a. Collect additional blood for the determination of morphine [2]

  b. Collect all bile for morphine and other alkaloidal analysis

  c. Take specimen of lung (one-half of one lung should be adequate)

2. Inhalation or solvent poisoning cases

  a. Tie off trachea

  b. Collect sample of bronchial air

  c. Collect entire lung and place in airtight container

3. Pesticide cases: take sample of fatty tissue (from abdominal wall or perinephric region)

4. Arsenic and heavy metal poisonings: take sample of hair, nails, and bone

5. Cholinesterase poisonings: take sample of brain and freeze

6. Pneumoconioses: take a sample of lung for analysis

---

 [2] Editors note: Communication with the laboratory analyst is essential. Different technics require different amounts of blood.

7. In instances of death from extensive trauma: take vitreous fluid for determination of alcohol
   a. Use syringe and 18 or 20 gauge needle
   b. Frequently available when other specimens are not because of extensive trauma

8. Embalmed cases
   a. Obtain sample of embalming fluid
   b. Take spleen
   c. Collect sample of marrow
   d. Obtain routine specimens

9. Exhumed bodies
   a. Know all available history before starting autopsy
   b. Do not hurry
   c. Obtain soil samples from above and beneath coffin
   d. Collect sample of any fluid found in coffin

10. Homicidal poisonings
    a. Very rare
    b. Take extra care to avoid cross-contamination during collection of specimens
    c. Prove the route of administration
       (1) Collect sample of air and sample of lung
       (2) Excise injection site including skin, fat, muscle; take control sample from contralateral site
       (3) remove entire gut by segments; measure contents
           (a) stomach
           (b) duodenum
           (c) jujunum
           (d) ileum
           (e) large bowel
    d. Extensive toxicologic studies are necessary; verify the drug by as many analytical methods as possible
    e. Rule out all other possible unrelated causes of death
    f. Take sample of hair, nails, bone, etc.
    g. Maintain chain of possession
    h. Eliminate possibility of container-originated contamination by checking similar containers for contaminants

Do's and Don'ts

1. Do a complete autopsy in every case, including microscopic examination, no matter how sure you are that it is a "straight forward case of barbiturate overdose."

2. If specimens are submitted for toxicologic examination, defer ("pend") the cause of death. Wait until complete toxicologic examination is finished to opine the cause of death.

3. Do not "sign out" death due to drugs without having before you all of the following:
   a. History or investigator's report
   b. Autopsy protocol
   c. All laboratory reports
   d. Microscopic reports
4. Double check to be sure that the toxicologist has analyzed for all drugs noted in the history
5. If low levels are found in the body fluids, consider
   a. Poly-pharmacy and look for more drugs
   b. Passage of time after ingestion with resulting metabolism of drug
6. Utilize all facts at your disposal in deciding upon a cause of death. If an individual survived in hospital 1 to 2 weeks do not indicate the cause of death as bronchopneumonia, but rather as bronchopneumonia following drug ingestion
7. Use generic names of drugs, not proprietary names
8. In ascribing manner of death, consider all factors
   a. Automatism "myth"
   b. Certain religions do not commit suicide "myth"
   c. Judge the poor as you would the rich who hire a vocal attorney
9. Know the most common poisons in your area (Alameda County— 1,000,000 population, 11-year span)
   a. Barbiturates
   b. Alcohol and barbiturate
   c. Intravenous narcotism
   d. Alcohol
   e. Cyanide
   f. Glutethimide
   g. Meprobamate
   h. Propoxyphene
   i. Salicylates
   j. Arsenic

178

Chapter XXIX
ALCOHOL

Arthur J. McBay, Ph.D.
Chief Toxicologist
Office of the Chief Medical Examiner
State of North Carolina
Chapel Hill, North Carolina

Introduction

The most common toxicologic analysis is that made for the quantitation of alcohol in biologic specimens. Alcohol is a poison and as such may be the direct cause of death when ingested in excessive amounts. Ingestion of 500 to 1000 ml. of 50 percent alcohol (100 proof liquor) in a short period of time (1 to 2 hours) may cause death by respiratory depression. Smaller amounts when combined with other respiratory depressants such as carbon monoxide, barbiturates, morphine, etc. may produce fatal results. For example, a blood alcohol concentration of 150 mg. percent with 0.5 mg. percent of rapid-acting barbiturate in the blood may be sufficient evidence to certify death by alcohol and barbiturates.* Significant amounts of alcohol are found in the blood of more than one-half of those whose deaths are either homicidal, suicidal, or accidental.

Alcohol is a contributory factor in many deaths because the impaired individual errs in judgment or more directly lacks control of his faculties. The largest, and probably best studied group, of alcohol-involved fatalities are those resulting from automobile crashes into fixed objects, other vehicles, and pedestrians. About 60 percent of the drivers killed in single-vehicle crashes are impaired by alcohol (100 mg. percent or more). The intoxicated individual may kill himself by falling, exposure to heat or cold, overdosing with drugs, being burnt in a fire or being exposed to noxious gases, trying to swallow too large a portion of food, aspiration, drowning, hanging, shooting, or stabbing.

Excessive amounts of alcohol produce irreversible brain and liver damage that can eventually prove to be fatal. "Moonshine" liquor generally contains ethyl alcohol produced under unsanitary conditions. It also may contain lead but rarely produces chronic lead intoxication.

---

* Editors note: The circumstances surrounding the death, history of long-term dosage with barbiturates and other details must be sought before such a death might be considered to be due to the additive effects of alcohol and barbiturates.

179

Other alcohols may be encountered; paint and other industrial solvents contain methyl alcohol and rubbing alcohol usually contains isopropyl alcohol. Formaldehyde contains methyl alcohol as a preservative.

Specimens

Adequate specimens should be submitted for alcohol determinations on all medicolegal deaths. The specimens should be obtained by a person who is aware of the problems produced by samples improperly obtained and knows how to avoid them. Samples should be obtained as soon as possible after death and before the body is embalmed or starts to decompose. Ethanol and other alcohols may be generated in the body after death and during storage of blood samples obtained at autopsy by fermentation of carbohydrates and proteins present in the blood.†

Samples should be obtained with a clean needle and syringe from the femoral or subclavian vessels or from the heart. Spinal fluid and vitreous humor make very good samples. Blood may be obtained from a chamber of the heart but fluid from the pericardial sac should not be used. Brain tissue is an excellent specimen for determination of alcohol. Diffusion of alcohol in the intact body should not affect any of the above specimens. Damage to organs and vessels should be evaluated in order to choose the proper site of collection or proper specimen. Each sample should be placed in a clean, dry container with sodium fluoride and should be refrigerated as soon as possible.

If the specimen is to be stored for an extended period before analysis, such as a week, it should be placed in a freezer. When blood is preserved with 1 percent sodium fluoride, no alcohol is generated for ten days when stored at room temperature. All containers should be properly identified. The chain of custody from the person obtaining the sample to the analyst must be not only known but documented. Adequate information should accompany the sample to inform the analyst of the examination requested, to properly identify the sample, and to provide historical data when needed.

The distribution of alcohol in various tissues varies directly with the amount in the tissue. With blood as 1.00, the average for brain is 1.17, for plasma, 1.16, for urine, 1.35, for liver, 0.91, and for blood clot, 0.77.[1]

Live Subjects

Occasionally the pathologist is concerned with testing blood, taken from a live person, for alcohol content. There is no special problem when blood is being drawn from a patient for diagnosis to guide treatment. In this instance the patient-physician privilege should prevail. The physician should not have to reveal the analytical results to the court.‡

---

† Editors note: Alcohol levels due to decomposition cannot be predicted with precision.

‡ Editors note: Depends upon the law of the particular State.

If the physician is subpoenaed, he should seek legal advice before he decides not to answer a question put to him in court. He should check state laws to see if physicians have any responsibility to report or not report habitual drinkers or alcoholics.

For traffic-related offenses, the operator should be tested for alcohol. In most States he must first be arrested, then asked to submit to a test of his breath or blood. A breath test properly performed with any of several of the electronic instruments available is capable of giving an accurate evaluation of the amount of alcohol in the blood. If a physician is asked to draw blood for legal purposes, he may do so or he may have an assistant or technician do so under his authority; he cannot be forced to do this. A non-alcoholic solution should be used to clean the area where the blood is to be drawn. The physician should not draw blood if the patient objects.§

It is preferable to draw the sample in the presence of a law enforcement officer and to give it to him to transport and to obtain the analysis. This may prevent the physician or technician from having to appear in court. If the physician or technician is to handle the sample, he should be responsible for the identification of that sample. In most States the sample can be sealed and sent by first class mail to the analyst. All those who handle the sample should be ready to testify to the identity of the sample.

A pathologist should be able to give an opinion on the sobriety of an individual observed by him. Table I could serve as a guide in forming an opinion. He should hesitate to offer an opinion on the sobriety of a person when that opinion is based solely on the blood alcohol level unless he has special knowledge in this field.

Methods for Analysis for Ethyl Alcohol

The methods employed in the analysis of the specimens depend on the type of sample, the resources available, the need for accuracy, and the need for specificity. An excellent reference covering the methods and other matters is readily available.[1] The simplest procedure is a "balloon-type" test. The use of this procedure requires little training, it is inexpensive, and the results are semi-quantitative. The electronic breath-testing instruments are relatively expensive, require training, but can give accurate, dependable results.

Specimens of blood may be screened for alcohol and other volatiles simply and inexpensively using a microdiffusion procedure.[5]

Distillation procedures and enzymatic alcohol dehydrogenase procedures[1] lack some specificity and therefore require additional tests to eliminate interference due to other alcohols and volatiles. For postmortem blood and other specimens, gas chromatography[1] offers the best

---

§ Editors note: Get legal advice!

TABLE I. Alcohol Concentration and Clinical Symptoms [2,3,4,||]

Blood Alcohol		Effects on Drinkers		Appearing Drunk	
(Percent)	(Mg%)	(Inexperienced)	(Experienced)	(Drinks#)	(Percent)
0–0.05	0–50	Not noticeable	Not noticeable	0–3	10
0.05–0.10	50–100	Slight	None to slight	3–6	34
0.10–0.15	100–150	Under the influence	Slight	6–9	64
0.15–0.20	150–200	Drunk	Under the influence	9–12	86
0.20–0.25	200–250	Drunk to very drunk	Influenced to drunk	12–15	96
0.25–0.30	250–300	Very drunk	Drunk to very drunk	15–18	99
0.30–0.40	300–400	Stupor to coma	Very drunk to stupor	18–21	
0.40–0.50	400–500	Comatose to death	Comatose to death	21–24	

Slight effects: Flushed face, dilated pupils; euphoria; loss of restraint.

Under the influence: Flushed face; dilated, sluggish pupils; euphoria; loss of restraint, carelessness and recklessness; incoordination; thickness of speech; stagger on sudden turning.

Drunk: Face flushed; pupils dilated and inactive; rapid movement of eyeballs; mood unstable; loss of restraint; clouding of intellect; thickness of speech; incoordination; staggering gait with reeling and lurching when called upon to make sudden turns.

Very drunk: Face flushed or pale. Pupils inactive, contracted, or dilated; mental confusion; gross incoordination; slurred speech; staggering, reeling gait; tendency to lurch and fall; vomiting.

|| Ounces of 100 proof liquor (50 percent alcohol) in a 150 pound person in a short period of time. Average person loses 18 mg. percent of alcohol per hour. The concentration of alcohol in the blood produced by a given quantity of alcohol varies with the type of drink, concentration of alcohol in the drink, the person's tolerance, the presence or absence of food in the stomach, the rate of drinking, and the weight of the individual.

In a study[2] where three double whiskies (5 ounces), one-half bottle of Burgundy, and two brandies were ingested in 2 and ½ hours with a meal, the blood reached an alcohol concentration of 0.06 percent. In another study where no food was consumed, a 0.08 percent blood alcohol concentration was produced by the ingestion of 6 ounces of whiskey in 2 hours or 4 pints (64 ounces) of beer in 1 and ¾ hours.

Editors note: Modified from Table II of le Roux and Smith.[4]

method for specificity although the initial cost is great and the method requires careful control.

Interpretation of Results

Lethal concentrations of alcohol in blood are usually greater than 250 mg. percent and may reach 500 to 600 mg. percent. Lower concentrations are significant especially when other central nervous system depressants are present or following prolonged coma or adverse physical defects.[7]

The concentration of alcohol in the dead body does not change until alcohol is formed as putrefaction commences.[6] Alcohol concentrations of up to about 200 mg. percent may develop during putrefaction and this will not necessarily indicate alcohol was present at death.** If alcohol is found in urine obtained post mortem the ingestion of alcohol prior to death is indicated. Drowning and burning per se usually do not affect the concentration of alcohol in tissues.

In addition to formaldehyde, embalming fluid contains methanol and also may contain ethanol and isopropanol. The embalming fluid may replace the blood. Alcohol concentrations found in embalmed bodies are unreliable.

Certification of Death

The certification of the cause and manner of death is difficult when alcohol is involved. Even in those cases where an excess of alcohol led directly to death, unless the word "poisoning" is used in the "cause" it is unlikely that alcohol as the cause of death will appear in vital statistics. The manner of death is an even greater problem. Does the person who drinks himself to death commit suicide or is his death accidental? Does a person drink to get up courage to commit suicide by other means or does his drunken condition mistakenly lead to an overdose of drug or some other misadventure? Unless other evidence to indicate suicide is present, the deaths of persons with high concentrations of alcohol should be considered accidental.††

Do's and Don'ts

1. Do use clean containers with adequate preservative.
2. Do know exact source of blood sample.
3. Do try to obtain samples before embalming or putrefaction.
4. Do properly mark and identify sample.
5. Do refrigerate samples while storing.

** Editors note: A 200 mg. percent blood or tissue alcohol level due to decomposition alone would be at the extreme high end of the spectrum. Levels to 100 mg. percent are much more apt to be encountered, and even this level is in the higher end of the spectrum.

†† Editors note: In many medical-legal jurisdictions, such deaths are certified as "manner of death: natural."

6. Do obtain antemortem sample if possible.
7. Do use sample from more than one area if postmortem diffusion is a possibility.
8. Do retain a frozen sample of about one ounce of liver (most toxicologic tests can be performed on this sample).
9. Do not take sample from pericardial sac.
10. Do not take sample from chest if this area has been pierced or broken.
11. Do not use contaminated needles, syringes, or containers.
12. Do not submit improperly identified samples.

References

1. Alcohol and the Impaired Driver: A Manual on the Medicolegal Aspects of Chemical Tests for Intoxication. American Medical Association, Chicago, 1970, 234 pp
2. Camps, FE, Robinson, A: Experiments to establish the amount of alcohol in the blood under social drinking conditions. Med Sci Law 8:153–160, 1968
3. Harger, RN, Hulpieu, HR: The pharmacology of alcohol, alcoholism. Edited by GN Thompson. Charles C Thomas, Springfield, 1956, pp 103–232
4. le Roux, CC, Smith, LS: Violent deaths and alcoholic intoxication. J Forensic Med, 11:131–147, 1964
5. McBay, AJ: Ethanol, Manual of Analytical Toxicology. Chemical Rubber Company, Cleveland, 1971, p 142
6. Plueckhahn, VD: The evaluation of autopsy blood alcohol levels. Med Sci Law 8:168–176, 1968
7. Saldeen, T, Johansson, O: The significance of chronic heart disease, fatty liver, and consumption of barbiturate and Librium on the tolerance of ethyl alcohol, as judged in a postmortem series. J Forensic Sci, 12:273–294, 1967

Chapter XXX
THERAPEUTIC MISADVENTURE

Charles S. Petty, M.D.
Chief Medical Examiner and Director
Southwestern Institute of Forensic Sciences
Dallas, Texas

What is a misadventure? According to Black's Law Dictionary, the definition is: "A mischance or accident; a casualty caused by the act of one person inflicting injury upon another. Homicide by 'misadventure' occurs when a man, doing a lawful act, without any intention of hurt, unfortunately kills another."

The American Heritage Dictionary of the English Language defines misadventure as "an instance of great misfortune; disaster."

Regardless of the "proper" definitions of misadventure, it is obvious to those who work in the field of forensic pathology, that the term is translated differently by physicians, attorneys, pathologists, hospital administrators, and vital statisticians. Perhaps no term used as frequently by all of the above, is interpreted so very differently.

To some, the term means malpractice; to others it means accident, with or without fault; still others argue that the term itself should be abolished. Little agreement has been reached.

Little has been written about therapeutic misadventure in the medical literature. Perhaps physicians would like to forget it, to sequester it into the subconscious. The British Association in Forensic Medicine held a symposium regarding therapeutic misadventure in 1959.[1] The lawyers point of view is expressed, to a degree, by Ficarra.[2] In this article the term "refers to a category of medical mishaps with implications of legal liability." Ficarra[2] also describes therapeutic misadventure as ". . . those new areas of possible medical negligence which are labeled 'therapeutic misadventure.' "

A little reflection will bring one to the conclusion that some fault or negligence upon the physicians' part may be inferred by reading the death certificate and finding upon it the term "therapeutic misadventure."

Allow me the liberty of example:

1A. A 25-year-old woman is treated for a severe infection by her physician. She is questioned about previous penicillin injections, and whether or not she had reactions to them. Yes, she had several treatments with intramuscular injections of penicillin with no reaction. The physician gives an injection of the drug and five minutes later, when on the way out of the office, she collapses and dies in anaphylaxis. This is clearly a therapeutic misadventure. No negligence would appear to attend the death.

1B. The same hypothetical infected woman under questioning stated she had a "bad reaction" the last time penicillin was used. She is unable to supply details of the reaction and the physician gives her an injection of the drug. She collapses and dies. This is clearly a therapeutic misadventure. There well may be negligence on the part of the treating physician.

2A. A 70-year-old man enters a dentist's office for extraction of his several remaining teeth under anesthesia with an intravenous agent. The dentist questions him in regard to his health and cardiovascular status. He admits to mild heart disease and hypertension. Because of this the dentist asks a physician to examine him and to stand by during the short procedure. The patient collapses and resuscitative procedures are to no avail. This is a therapeutic misadventure with a very low potential of negligence.

2B. This is the same hypothetical man who admits to mild heart disease and hypertension. Without further examination the dentist carries out both anesthesia and extractions. The patient collapses. The dentist is unable to render adequate resuscitative measures and to revive the patient. Another therapeutic misadventure. The negligence potential is very high.

The death certificates would be identical:

Cause of death—Death during anesthesia for dental extractions.
Other significant conditions contributing to death: heart disease.
Manner of death—"Therapeutic misadventure," therefore accident.
Some might want to certify death as natural due to heart disease.

It is this latter possibility "manner of death, natural (heart disease)" as the evaluation of the death by the dentist that would perhaps prevent a report of this death to the medicolegal officer and would, therefore, make it impossible to properly assess the number of individuals who die in dentists' offices.

The term "therapeutic misadventure" certainly does not mean, or even imply medical negligence either of a civil or a criminal nature. Perhaps it does serve as a screen to separate instances of "zero negligence potential" from "possible negligence potential." In this way the term may prove to be of use in tagging or flagging cases in medicolegal offices.

Therapeutic misadventure may be subdivided into "therapeutic" (when treatment is being given), "diagnostic" (where diagnosis only is the objective at the time), and "experimental" (where the patient has agreed to serve as a subject in an experimental study). Physicians, surgeons, nurses, respiratory therapists, pharmacists, and many paramedical individuals may precipitate a therapeutic misadventure.

The medicolegal officer has the duty to properly certify the death and usually finds himself in a position where he cannot assign fault. Furthermore, the death certificate is not the proper instrument upon which to detail possible or potential negligence. This is for other officials and legal agencies to decide. The certifier of the death has many duties: to the law, next of kin, medical societies, law enforcement agencies, district attorneys, etc., etc. It is his duty to indicate on the death certificate the best analysis of all he knows about the cause of death. If the death is, indeed, a therapeutic misadventure, then it must be stated and if so the manner of death must be indicated as "accident."

In investigating a possible therapeutic misadventure, the forensic pathologist must interview all of those involved: the surgeon, anethesiologist, nurse, pharmacist, etc., etc. It is amazing how differently the several members of an operating team view the same case.

It may be necessary to seek the services of different experts to study the circumstances of death. In an operating room death this may involve other surgeons, anesthesiologists, nurses, transfusion specialists, electrical engineers, etc. It would be important to impound and keep from further use anesthesia machines, used blood containers, and all the paraphernalia of the modern surgery. The dead patient should be left as he was at death: all tubes still in place. No postmortem removal of organs for transplantation (mini-autopsy) should be permitted. All records, charts, recordings, etc. should be available for review. This type of investigation is the most difficult forensic challenge of all to meet.

To accomplish all of this, early reporting of the death is essential, followed by active participation of the medicolegal officer in the investigation. Cooperation between all parties based upon mutual confidence and trust is essential. Confidentiality of all records must be maintained.

Simply because the death is investigated by the medicolegal officer does not imply that there is a fault on the part of the physician (hospital or others) that an accident took place, or that cause for malpractice action exists. It is most important that the forensic pathologist or medicolegal officer investigate each apparent therapeutic misadventure thoroughly, document the findings and be prepared to present the accumulated data to many different persons, each with his own ends to pursue.

Do's and Don'ts

1. Do investigate each possible instance of "therapeutic misadventure" completely and without becoming an advocate for any cause.
2. Do use specialists and experts in all fields to further investigate those areas not completely familiar to you.
3. Do insist that you, the pathologist, be advised of the death very early in the investigation so that steps can be taken to prevent

alteration or obliteration of useful evidence by manipulation of the body, removal of tracheostomy and/or other tubes and hasty repairs or malfunctioning equipment before you, an impartial examiner, can get to body and machines.

4. Do insist upon reviewing all records related to the dead patient. Indeed, it may be necessary to review serial records of the pharmacy, blood bank, clinical laboratory and others so as to view the deceased person's treatment in proper perspective.

5. Do not, without adequate, conscientious investigation, prepare a premature, hastily-conceived report of what may be an extremely complicated death situation. Better by far to delay the death certification than to move too rapidly.

Do not make premature statements to the press or to others for press release until the investigation is complete.

References

1. British Association in Forensic Medicine: Symposium: therapeutic misadventure. J Forensic Med 7:177–224, 1959

2. Ficarra, BJ: Therapeutic misadventure, Legal Medicine Annual: 1971. Edited by CH Wecht. Appleton-Century-Crofts, New York, 1971, pp. 389–413

Chapter XXXI
THE MOTOR VEHICLE CRASH: MEDICOLEGAL INVESTIGATION

Charles S. Petty, M.D.
Chief Medical Examiner and Director
Southwestern Institute of Forensic Sciences
Dallas, Texas

and

William G. Eckert, M.D.
Deputy Coroner, Sedgwick County
Wichita, Kansas

Introduction

This chapter is concerned with the special forensic problems associated with deaths related to motor vehicle crashes. An outline designed to alert the pathologist to the various medicolegal ramifications pertaining to deaths involving motor vehicles is presented.

The major categories of persons found dead where motor vehicles have or may have had a role in death include:

1. The driver
2. The passenger
3. The pedestrian
4. Do not know (1 or 2 above)
5. Do not know: body lying on berm or near road
6. Individual precipitated (accidentally or deliberately) from motor vehicle

The first problem faced by the pathologist (and the medicolegal investigator) is to properly categorize the individual whose body is the subject of examination.

1. The driver
   a. The only occupant of the vehicle
   b. By position in the vehicle upon discovery (possible only if the vehicle has not rolled over or impacted so that the driver and the passenger could have transposed positions)
   c. By establishment of:
      (1) Pedal or dimmer switch imprints on shoe soles
      (2) Fiber-clothing match

189

(3) Blood stain-blood type match
(4) Hair match
(5) Fingerprints on steering wheel
(6) Specific injuries caused by objects so positioned in the vehicle that a passenger could not have been so injured

    d. Witness to crash having no vested interest in the crash
       (1) Beware of the witness who was in the vehicle—frequently claims he was not the driver when the other occupant is dead
       (2) Rarely a witness involved in the crash may have no true recollection of it: post-traumatic amnesia

2. The passenger
    a. By position in vehicle upon discovery (possibly only if vehicle has not rolled over or otherwise impacted so that the driver and the passenger could have transposed positions)
    b. By establishment of:
       (1) Fiber-clothing match
       (2) Blood stain-blood type match
       (3) Hair match
       (4) Specific injuries caused by objects so positioned in the vehicle that the driver could not have been so injured
    c. Witness to the crash having no vested interest in the crash
       (1) Beware of a witness who was in the vehicle
       (2) Rarely a witness involved in the crash may have true post-traumatic amnesia

3. The pedestrian
    a. Known or acknowledged pedestrian, confirmed by:
       (1) Injuries which fit a predicted pattern
          (a) Point of impact
          (b) "Bumper" fractures
          (c) "Moving head" type of coup-contracoup cerebral contusions
          (d) Specific injuries that fit striking objects (patterned abrasions, contusions, lacerations)
       (2) Cross-transfer of physical evidence fits prediction
          (a) Transfer of grease, paints, or broken glass from striking objects to victim
          (b) Transfer of blood, hair, fibers, tissue to motor vehicle
          (c) Patterned imprints of fabric in paint or dust on motor vehicle
          (d) Dents in metal at impact points that fit with the pedestrian's size and/or injuries

(3) Evidence from a witness having no vested interest in the crash
    (a) Avoid the witness who was in the striking automobile
    (b) Remember more than one vehicle may strike the same pedestrian (this is particularly true in the high-density traffic situations of today)
  b. Probable pedestrian based upon:
    (1) Injury pattern
    (2) Transfer of physical evidence probably originating from a motor vehicle to the body
    (3) Location of the body in the road, on the berm, or near a roadway
4. Do not know whether driver or passenger
  a. Confusing cross-transfer of evidence between automobile and occupant
  b. No injury pattern clearly indicating whether driver or passenger
  c. Roll over, extreme impact, ejection of occupants
  d. No (or unreliable) witness
5. Do not know: body lying on the road, or berm, or near the road
  a. Rarely may have no external injuries and be a motor vehicle-pedestrian accident victim
  b. Injuries may be inapparent (fracture of cervical vertebrae) unless special pains are taken at autopsy to demonstrate
  c. May be no motor vehicle to examine for transfer of evidence (hit-and-run situation)
  d. May actually be a mistaken impression by motor vehicle driver that he struck body
  e. Person may already have been dead and was run over by motor vehicle or thought by driver to have been run over
6. Individual precipitated (accidentally or deliberately) from motor vehicle
  a. Accidental loss of individual from motor vehicle
    (1) Loss may not be at once recognized
      (a) Especially from back of truck or trailer
      (b) Darkness and traffic plus road conditions may contribute
    (2) Loss may be recognized at once but traffic may not permit rapid stop
      (a) Following vehicle(s) may run over or strike the precipitated individual
      (b) Driver of following vehicle may think he has struck the precipitated individual
  b. Individual deliberately precipitated from the motor vehicle
    (1) Usually dumped in darkness or in untraveled area

191

      (2) High level of alcohol or drugs, or dead or incapacitated by injury

      (3) Pattern of injury may not fit with the scene where found

7. Variations in the manner of death
   a. Accident
   b. Accident-natural disease combinations (trauma in itself insufficient to account for death)
   c. Suicide
      (1) Crash (usually single occupant) into fixed object
      (2) Pedestrian walking or running in front of motor vehicle
      (3) Other (additional) methods employed for suicide:
          (a) Drugs plus "accident"
          (b) Slashing of wrists plus "accident"
          (c) Gunshot wounds plus "accident"
   d. Homicide
      (1) Deliberate running-down of victim or automobile
      (2) Situational: failure to stop and render aid (hit-and-run)

8. Cause of the "accident"
   a. Natural disease processes
      (1) Presence provable but exact importance questionable
          (a) History of epilepsy in some cases:
              Look for epileptogenic lesion in the brain
              Analyze blood for the presence of suppressive drugs
          (b) Disease of the heart and blood vessels
              Arteriosclerotic heart disease
              Rheumatic heart disease
              Hypertensive heart disease
              Dissecting aneurysm of the aorta
              Abdominal aortic aneurysm
              Syphilitic heart disease
          (c) Congenital aneurysm of the cerebral vessels
          (d) Brain tumor
          (e) Diabetes
              Hypoglycemia
              Insulin shock
          (f) Poor sight or hearing as a result of disease, post trauma, or aging
      (2) Presence not provable
          (a) Epilepsy in some cases
          (b) Heart disease and associated problems:
              Angina
              Stokes-Adams attacks
              Wolff-Parkinson-White syndrome
              Carotid sinus hypersensitivity

192

Sudden disturbing arrhythmias
Hypertensive encephalopathy
    (c) Senility
    (d) Mental (emotional) disease
  b. Many other important entities, including:
    (1) Alcohol
    (2) Carbon monoxide
    (3) Alcohol or carbon monoxide plus barbiturates, tranquilizers or other drugs
    (4) Menstruation
  c. Suicide
  d. Other
    (1) Mechanical failure
    (2) Highway: poor design and maintenance
  f. Evidence of witness
    (1) Watch for bias
    (2) The witness who was inside the crash vehicle vs. the witness who observes the crash from outside the vehicle
9. Special Situations
  a. Seat belt
    (1) Contribution to safety
    (2) Contribution to injury
    (3) Contribution to accident
  b. Twice-hit pedestrian
  c. The person prone or supine on the road
    (1) Sleeping
    (2) Drunk or drugged
    (3) Incapacitated due to disease
    (4) Confused

Do's and Don'ts

1. Do not do an autopsy until you know the circumstances of the crash (or case). Remember: more may be lost by rushing to perform an immediate autopsy than by waiting a few hours to allow time for the investigational information to reach you. A waiting period is also useful so as to be able to contact the family and to make them aware of the medicolegal aspects which may not be apparent to them at first.

2. Do photograph and diagram all external evidence of injury. The solution to many insurance problems may depend upon this. Documentation of the appearance of the body is the key to problem solving, especially if the court cannot hear the case for many months, or even years.

3. Do get a copy of the police investigation reports and photographs. Reference to these may save much embarrassment at a later time. Many crash victims are moved quickly to permit possible resuscita-

tion, or to prevent the curious from blocking traffic and endangering lives. The pathologist, because of the press of other duties, may not be able to visit the scene. The crash vehicle, however, may remain in a police pound or repair yard, untouched, for a considerable time, long enough to permit the pathologist to examine it. Even a retrospective examination may be of great use in correlation of vehicle and injuries.

4. Do get the law enforcement or medicolegal investigators to secure the control pedals from the vehicle (to compare with the shoes of occupants) if any question develops regarding the possibility of a suicidal crash or determining who was driving at the time of the crash.

5. Do not be satisfied to "just perform the autopsy." An autopsy not correlated with investigational and other facts is a waste of expensive time.

6. Do not take anything at face value. Remember that the crash investigators may be inexperienced, and worse, may have little imagination. The pathologist may be in an excellent position to correlate all of the information regarding the crash.

7. Do be a collector. Collect, preserve, and retain anything that might possibly establish a correlation between the pedestrian victim and the offending vehicle: hair, blood, clothing, paint or other foreign particles, grease, glass, etc. Comparison of these objects *may* not be possible, but without them, no comparison *will* be possible!

References

The following are useful references. The older references have stood the test of time. The influence which alcohol has on automobile drivers and the "crash cause" is unquestioned. The role of drugs in causing motor vehicle crashes is only now being recognized.

Motor Vehicle Crashes—General

1. Brinkhous, KM: Accident Pathology, Proceedings of an International Conference. Washington, DC, June 6–8, 1968. Government Printing Office, Washington, DC, 1968, 249 pp

2. Eckert, WG, Kemmerer, WT, Chetta, N: The traumatic pathology of traffic accidents. J Forensic Sci 4:309–329, 1959

3. Huelke, D, Gikas, P: Causes of death in traffic accidents. JAMA 203:1100–1107, 1968

4. Kulowski, J: Crash Injuries. Charles C Thomas, Springfield, 1960, 1080 pp

5. Peterson, BJ, Petty, CS: Sudden natural death among automobile drivers. J Forensic Sci 7:274–285, 1962

6. Roberts, HJ: The Causes, Ecology and Prevention of Traffic Accidents. Charles C Thomas, Springfield, 1971, 1016 pp

Trace Evidence in Motor Vehicle Crashes

1. Huelke, D, Gikas, P: Investigations of fatal automobile accidents from the forensic standpoint. J Forensic Sci 11:474–484, 1966

2. Petty, CS, Smith, RA, Hutson, TA: The value of shoesole imprints in automobile crash investigations. J Police Sci Admin 1:1–10, 1973

3. Stratton, F: Miscellaneous trace evidence in automobile cases. J Forensic Sci 3:73–83, 1958

Alcohol Drugs and Driving

1. AMA Committee on Medicolegal Problems: Alcohol and the Impaired Driver. American Medical Association, Chicago, 1968, 234 pp
2. Forney, RB, Hughes, FW: Combined Effects of Alcohol and Other Drugs. Charles C Thomas, Springfield, 1968, 124 pp
3. Kay, S: Blood alcohol levels and fatal traffic accidents. Biol Assoc Med P Rico 61: 244–249, 1969
4. Polacsek, E, Barnes, T, Turner, N, et al: Interaction of Alcohol and Other Drugs. Second edition. Addiction Research Foundation, Toronto, 1972, 561 pp
5. Waller, JA: Holiday drinking and highway fatalities. JAMA 206:2692–2697, 1968
6. Waller, A: Drugs and highway crashes. JAMA 215:1477–1482, 1971

Chapter XXXII

A FORENSIC LIBRARY FOR A NON-FORENSIC PATHOLOGIST

Charles S. Petty, M.D.
Chief Medical Examiner of Dallas County
Director, Institute of Forensic Sciences
Dallas, Texas

Frequently I am asked to suggest the "best" textbooks available in forensic pathology. At other times the question takes the form of "please suggest a library for me—I'm going to an area where I will practice general pathology but will be expected to carry out medicolegal autopsies."

Of course, every book printed offers something; some more than others. There is no "best" book, and anyone who ventures to select one book and not another opens himself to considerable criticism. I would offer, regardless of criticism, the following nineteen books as the nucleus of a forensic library. Some are old, out of print classics; others are brand new. Some are excellent throughout; others are spotty and present sections both good and bad, with the former outweighing the latter.

1. **General Forensic Pathology**
   a. Spitz, W. U., and Fisher, R. S. *Medicolegal Investigation of Death*. Springfield: Charles C. Thomas, 1973, 536 pp.
   The editors do not claim that theirs is a "compleat" textbook. For the most part it is easy to read and well-illustrated. Those who have written chapters were well selected.
   b. Adelson, L. *The Pathology of Homicide*. Springfield: Charles C. Thomas, 1974, 976 pp.
   Written entirely by one who knows the King's English as well as forensic pathology. Brand new and a textbook, I believe, destined to become a classic.
   c. Polson, C. J. *The Essentials of Forensic Medicine*. Second edition. Springfield: Charles C. Thomas, 1965, 600 pp.
   Some sections of this general textbook are superb. Some of the included material deals with matters English and is of little interest to those in the United States. Despite these drawbacks a worthwhile inclusion in the library.

196

d. Camps, F. E. *Gradwohl's Legal Medicine.* Second edition. Bristol: Wright, 1968, 740 pp.

This is also an English textbook. Like the first edition, edited by Dr. Gradwohl, this work is excellent in some areas and totally neglects others. However, its advantages earn it a place in this listing.

e. Brinkhous, K. M. *Accident Pathology.* Washington, DC: Government Printing Office, 1970, 249 pp.

Written by the many participants of a 1968 conference regarding accident pathology. A good overview of trauma.

f. Krogman, W. M. *The Human Skeleton in Forensic Medicine.* Springfield: Charles C. Thomas, 1962, 337 pp.

Perhaps "not all you need to know" about physical anthropology, but an excellent reference to help with the determination of the age, sex, race, and stature of skeletal remains!

g. Ludwig, J. *Current Methods of Autopsy Practice.* Philadelphia: W. B. Saunders, 1972, 356 pp.

Not really a forensic textbook. The book, however, can be a great aid to the pathologist in the conduct of a medicolegal autopsy.

2. Forensic Sciences and Relationship to the Law

a. Moenssens, A. A.; Moses, R. E.; and Inbau, F. E. *Scientific Evidence in Criminal Cases.* Mineola, New York: Foundation Press, 1973, 604 pp.

Written primarily for attorneys, but well worth owning. It will give the pathologist a new view of his own type of work as well as that of other forensic scientists.

3. Legal Aspects of Forensic Medicine

a. Holder, A. R. *Medical Malpractice Law.* New York: Wiley, 1975, 561 pp.

Full of "capsule cases" to illustrate problems in medical negligence with a thread of explanation to bind them all together.

b. Waltz, J. R., and Inbau, F. E. *Medical Jurisprudence.* New York: Macmillan, 1971, 398 pp.

A short text regarding medical jurisprudence and allied matters. Excellent for helping to prepare lectures for medical students.

c. Horsley, J. E., and Carlova, J. *Testifying in Court: The Advanced Course.* Oradell, NJ: Medical Economics, 1972, 104 pp.

A short guide on "how to." Great for those who are apprehensive about courtroom appearances.

4. The following listed are older classics. Alas! They are out of print. Should you happen across them, keep them, study them, and learn how little forensic problems have altered since the last edition of Peterson, Haines, and Webster was published in 1923.

a. Peterson, F.; Haines, W. S.; and Webster, R. W. *Legal Medicine and Toxicology,* Volumes I and II. Second edition. Philadelphia: W. B. Saunders, 1923, 1196 pp and 1072 pp.

b. Moritz, A. R. *The Pathology of Trauma.* Second edition. Philadelphia: Lea and Febiger, 1954, 414 pp.

c. Gonzales, T. A.; Vance, M.; and Helpern, M., et al. *Legal Medicine.* Second edition. New York: Appleton-Century-Crofts, 1954, 1349 pp.

5. A Word About Forensic Periodicals

Much of the information of forensic importance is published in nonforensic literature. It would require more time than anyone has available to scan all journals which publish articles of forensic interest.

The more "pure" forensic journals written in English are listed below:

a. **American.**

(1) *Journal of Forensic Sciences.*

Published quarterly. This is the official organ of the American Academy of Forensic Sciences. Subscription office: 1916 Race Street, Philadelphia, Pennsylvania 19103.

(2) *Legal Medicine Annual:* 1969, 1970, 1971, 1972, 1973, 1974. Edited by C. H. Wecht.

Published annually by Appleton-Century-Crofts, New York, Part legal, part medical; articles by both scientists and attorneys.

(3) *International Microfilm Journal of Legal Medicine.* Edited by Milton Helpern, University Microfilms, 300 North Zeeb Road, Ann Arbor, Michigan 48103.

(4) INFORM. Edited by William G. Eckert, MD.

Published by the International Reference Organization in Forensic Medicine. Subscription office: St. Francis Hospital, Wichita, Kansas 67214.

(5) *Journal of Legal Medicine (American College of Legal Medicine).* Edited by William H. L. Dornette. GMT Medical Information Systems, Inc., 777 Third Avenue, New York 10017.

American Journal of Law and Medicine.

The official publication of the American Society of Law and Medicine. Subscription office: 454 Brookline Avenue, Boston, Massachusetts 02215.

(6) *Medico-legal Bulletin.*

Obtainable from the Office of the Chief Medical Examiner, Virginia, 9 North 14th Street, Richmond, Virginia 23219.

(7) *The Forensic Science Gazette.* Edited by Vincent J. M. Di-Maio, MD. Subscription office: Post Office Box 35728, Dallas, Texas 75235.

b. **English**
 (1) *Medicine, Science and the Law.*
The official journal of the British Academy of Forensic Sciences. Write: John Wright and Sons, Ltd, Medicine, Science and the Law, 42-44 Triangle West, Bristol BS8, 1 EX, England.
 (2) *Journal of Forensic Science Society.*
Published by the Forensic Science Society and includes the Proceedings of the California Association of Criminalists. Subscription office: The Forensic Science Society, 107 Fenchurch Street, London 5 JB, England.
 (3) *Medico-legal Journal.*
Edited by Gavin Thurston. Heffers Printers Ltd, Cambridge, England.
c. **Other foreign (but printed in English).**
Forensic Science (supplanting the Journal of Forensic Medicine). Elsevier Sequoia SA, Post Office Box 851, 1001 Lausanne 1, Switzerland.

A logical extension of the Forensic Pathology library is a set of books relating to toxicology. Most of the toxicology textbooks and monographs deal with methodology. However, the forensic pathologist is more concerned with the interpretation of toxicologic data than in how to carry out analyses for toxic substances.

The books listed below are of great use to any practicing forensic pathologist:

(1) *AMA Drug Evaluations.* Second Edition. AMA, Department of Drugs. Acton, Massachusetts: Publishing Sciences Group, Inc., 1973, 1030 pp.

(2) Thienes, C. H., and Haley, T. J. *Clinical Toxicology.* Philadelphia: Lea and Febiger, 1972, 459 pp.

(3) Goodman, L. S., and Gilman, A. *The Pharmacological Basis of Therapeutics.* Fourth edition. New York: Macmillan, 1970, 1794 pp.

(4) Clarke, E. G. C. *Isolation and Identification of Drugs,* Volume 1. London: The Pharmaceutical Press, 1969, 870 pp.

(5) Clarke, E. G. C. *Isolation and Identification of Drugs,* Volume 2. London: The Pharmaceutical Press, 1975, 387 pp.

To help in interpretation, the following list of "maximum therapeutic levels" and "minimum lethal levels" of commonly encountered toxins is included. This was compiled by the Chief Toxicologist of the Southwestern Institute of Forensic Sciences at Dallas (Texas). Although these "levels" may not be taken as absolute, they at least are in perspective and in the correct order of magnitude.

Therapeutic and Toxic Concentrations of Common Drugs and Poisons
James C. Garriott, Ph.D.

	ORAL DOSE mg	MAXIMUM THERAPEUTIC LEVELS Blood Level mg%	MINIMUM LETHAL LEVELS Blood mg%
Acetaminophen	325–2600	3.00	——
Amitriptyline	50 t.i.d.	0.008	0.50
Amphetamine	5–30	0.002–0.010	(0.10)
Arsenic	"Normal"	0.007	0.07
Barbiturates:			
Slow Acting—			
(Phenobarbital)	600	2.50	5.00
Rapid Acting—			
(Secobarbital)	100–200	0.20–0.40	1.00
Boron	"Normal"	0.08	4.00
Bromides	"Normal"	5.00	100.0
Carbon monoxide	"Normal" smoker	7% carboxy-hemoglobin saturation (maximum—13%)	50% carboxy-hemoglobin saturation
Caffeine	300	0.50	15.0
Chloral hydrate	1000	1.00*	10.0*
Chlordiazepoxide	150/d	1.00	3.00
	30	0.10–0.20	——
Chlorpromazine	1000/d	0.10	1.00
Chlorpropamide	100–250/d	3.00–14.00	——
Chloroquine	300	0.15	——
Chlorzoxazone	1000	1.00–2.00	——
Codeine	15	0.003	0.20
Cyanide	——	——	0.50
Diazepam	40/d	0.10	2.00
Digoxin	0.25/d	0.7–2.0 ng/ml	4.0 ng/ml
Digitoxin	0.20/d	10.5–30 ng/ml	34 ng/ml
Diphenylhydantoin	600	1.00–2.00	5.00–10.00
Diphenhydramine	400	0.10	1.00
Ethanol	1 oz. (2 oz. whiskey or 2 bottles beer)	50.0	400.0
Ethchlorvynol	200	0.20	10.00
	1000	1.40	
Fluoride	"Normal"	0.01	0.30
Glutethimide	1000	0.75	2.00
Halothane	1% anesthetic gas	15.00	——
Hexachlorophene	None	None	1.00
Imipramine	300/d	0.06	0.20
Lead	Normal Max.	0.06	(0.10)
Lidocaine	500–100 mg (iv)	0.20–1.00	——
Meperidine	100	0.20	0.50
Meprobamate	400	0.50	5.00

Therapeutic and Toxic Concentrations of Common Drugs and Poisons (Continued):

	ORAL DOSE mg	MAXIMUM THERAPEUTIC LEVELS Blood Level mg%	MINIMUM LETHAL LEVELS Blood mg%
Mercury	Normal Max.	0.002	0.300
Methadone	(Tolerant) 40–120 (Non Tolerant)	0.01	0.10
Methamphetamine	5–10	0.010	0.10
Methaqualone	500	0.50	2.00
Methyprylon	300	1.00	3.00
Morphine	10(iv)	0.008	0.05
Nicotine	"Normal" smoker	0.030	0.50
Orphenadrine	60	——	0.40
Paraldehyde	10 ml (im)	7.70	50.00
Pentazocine	50	0.05	0.30
Phenylbutazone	——	5.00–15.00	——
Primidone	250–1500/d	0.20–1.90	——
Procainamide	1000–4000/d	0.40–0.80	1.20
Propoxyphene	130	0.012	0.20
Quinidine	600 mg	0.30–0.60	——
Quinine	1000	0.20	1.00
Salicylate	1000	10.00	50.00
Strychnine	——	——	0.20
Thioridazine	50–800/d	0.23	0.50

* Trichloroethanol
d = day
iv = intravenous
im = intramuscular

References

1. Baselt, R, Wright, J, Cravey, RH: Therapeutic and toxic concentrations of more than 100 toxicologically significant deaths in blood, plasma, or serum: a tabulation. Clin Chem 21:44–62, 1975
2. Garriott, JC: Personal observations
3. McBay, AJ: Personal communication, 1973
4. Vesell, ES, Passananti, GT: Utility of clinical chemical determinations of drug concentrations in biological fluids. Clin Chem 17:851–866, 1971

I hesitate to indicate textbooks in police science and investigation. However, I would suggest as a most provocative article the following which deals with "eyeball" witnesses: reading this may change your mind relative to "investigational" information.

1. Buckhout, R: Eyewitness Testimony. Scientific American 231:23–31, 1974

U.S. GOVERNMENT PRINTING OFFICE : 1979 O - 288-953